ONE HOUR POWER DIET

ONE HOUR
POWER DIET

One Hour Can Change Your Life
...and It Only Takes Minutes

CLIFF THOMAS, MD

New York

ONE HOUR POWER DIET
One Hour Can Change Your Life and It Only Takes Minutes

Published in New York, New York, by Morgan James Publishing. Morgan James and The Entrepreneurial Publisher are trademarks of Morgan James, LLC. www.MorganJamesPublishing.com

The Morgan James Speakers Group can bring authors to your live event. For more information or to book an event visit The Morgan James Speakers Group at www.TheMorganJamesSpeakersGroup.com.

Shelfie

A **free** eBook edition is available with the purchase of this print book.

CLEARLY PRINT YOUR NAME ABOVE IN UPPER CASE

Instructions to claim your free eBook edition:
1. Download the Shelfie app for Android or iOS
2. Write your name in **UPPER CASE** above
3. Use the Shelfie app to submit a photo
4. Download your eBook to any device

ISBN 978-1-63047-473-7 paperback
ISBN 978-1-63047-464-5 eBook
Library of Congress Control Number:
2014960163

Editor:
William Brohaugh
Wbrohaugh@yahoo.com

Interior Design by:
Bonnie Bushman
bonnie@caboodlegraphics.com

In an effort to support local communities and raise awareness and funds, Morgan James Publishing donates a percentage of all book sales for the life of each book to Habitat for Humanity Peninsula and Greater Williamsburg.

Get involved today, visit
www.MorganJamesBuilds.com

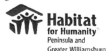

Habitat
for Humanity
Peninsula and
Greater Williamsburg
Building Partner

Table of Contents

Introduction   ix

You're the only one that can judge how you feel, what makes you feel better, and what makes you feel worse. Scientists have spent tremendous effort trying to measure energy production in relationship to food, when the way to measure how much energy you get from eating is simply asking yourself how you feel and then measuring it on your personal scale.

Chapter 1: Overcoming Weight-Loss "Infobesity"   1

Almost every day we hear, "This study proves X." Later, we hear, "This study proves the opposite of X." This overload of information leaves us feeling confused. The only way you will have long-term weight-loss success is to stick to a path that works for you. Here's how to find that path through the clutter of weight-loss "expertise."

Chapter 2: Experience Is the Foundation of Expertise   9
As with every important challenge in life, when facing the rewards of changing your life and rediscovering the real you, look for eating-right advice from experts that have experience and great mentors. The author of this book has both. Here he explains why he can guide you in looking beyond the marketing hype and using your energy to change wisely.

Chapter 3:   You Are the Goal—and You Are the Solution   20
The best barometer for what works is you. The solution is you. There's nothing in this book you don't already know, at least intuitively. But you may not be applying what you know. You may not even be aware of what you know— and awareness is the key to all change. This book brings awareness to what you already know as true and what will work for you.

Chapter 4:   Getting Real About Eating Healthier and Losing Weight   26
There's been too much questionable science around food and its affect on the body. For instance, the traditional food pyramid has a misconceived foundation, and it's time for a new pyramid—the pyramid of personal knowledge.

Chapter 5:   Your Food, Your Life—Step by Step   30
The process of growing healthier—and lighter—begins when you learn how your mind and body responds to the food you eat. When you know that, you will know

what food nourishes your body while allowing you to lose pounds.

Chapter 6: Committing to Changing Your Habits—Are You Ready? 45
The #1 challenge to long-term weight loss and healthy-eating success is committing to a process of change—for the rest of your life. Until you're ready to commit, you're wasting your time and energy. Here's how to take that critical next step—and to take it in the most effective way possible.

Chapter 7: Changing Eating Habits Made Easier 48
Developing new habits doesn't happen overnight. Some say it takes 21 days to change a habit, but I like to think in terms of chipping away and getting better and better. You must have a clear emotional view of where you want to be and not focus on how long it may take. Learn to love the journey—here's how to develop realistic expectations.

Chapter 8: Why You Eat What You Eat 57
Though many diets advise what you should eat, the first question to answer is Why do you eat? We eat for nutrients, we eat for pleasure, and we eat to satisfy dysfunctional needs. Understanding those reasons, we can adjust our eating patterns. Here's how.

Chapter 9: Tools for Success—Changing Your Eating Habits, 69 Changing Your Life
Your Life Pathways to feel-good success: "bite-sized" but critical strategies for changing your eating habits, changing your life, and becoming the real you.

Chapter 10: Pitfalls to Success and How to Leap Over Them   93
The challenges to becoming healthier and losing weight are persistent, and though they're difficult to overcome, they can be conquered. To avoid the pitfalls, people must rely on the only true measure of health and weight-loss success: their own bodies.

Chapter 11: Becoming Your Own Nutrition Expert   107
Experts can contribute valuable advice and insights into the nutritional value of foods and how your body uses them. But the key expert remains you.

About the Author   115

Introduction

"If you want to change your life, change your food."
– Yogi Bhajan

One hour per meal can change your life.

And it only takes minutes.

Have you awakened from a long, deep sleep to a body you don't recognize as you?

So what happened over all that time? Years and years of mindless food choices, eating on the run, eating fast food and eating fast, showing love through food, the "one more bite" mentality, and the idea that we can dump any food into our gastric system and wake up feeling good—that's what happened. And you know this.

It doesn't help that we live in a food-rich environment, and that our food has changed and is full of chemical additives.

After years of unconscious eating, we walk into a gym and hire a trainer and expect them to guide us to fast, sustainable weight loss within weeks. We start some weight loss fad and expect it to be the magic answer.

And we keep trying to play the game over and over. Then comes the feeling of blame. Don't waste your time and energy blaming yourself. It will beat you up. Begin with recognizing what does not work and contrast that with what does work. Then when you recognize what works and a day comes along where you did not do well, ask yourself how you can do better tomorrow. There are no mistakes, if we learn from them.

When it comes to getting healthy and losing weight, information and advice coming from the experts is confusing, conflicting, and often misleading. Most of that advice is based on poor science about a very complex and poorly understood system—our gut and our "gut brain."

What makes this problem worse is that the sheer volume of information about nutrition and health and weight loss is enormous. We're bombarded with what my colleague Sam Horn calls "infobesity." Too much weighty information about the topic of too much physical weight. How ironic is that? And despite year after year of receiving even good advice, we seem to be in the same place, or getting worse.

The problems are compounded by the fact we're all different, with different tastes, food choices, cultural traditions, and food sensitivities.

In the first chapter of *The One Hour Power Diet*, we take a closer look at "what we are doing," because what we're doing isn't working. Understanding what isn't working allows us to move on to what *does* work.

At the end of this introduction, I'll share a simple, powerful tool that does work—one hour power, a method that takes only minutes.

Much of "what we are doing" are poor indicators of success and create false expectations.

The problem with beliefs like a 30-day weight-loss plan is sustainable, or that a measurement like calories informs us about food energy, is that they create false expectations. Expectations make us believe that by doing some action we'll get a certain result. When we give that misleading action our energy and we don't see the results we expect, we want to quit.

Things that make us want to quit include:

- Poor indicators of success
- False expectations
- Perception that the method is too difficult
- Life and its day-to-day obstacles
- Unsustainable methods
- Resistance to change

We will benefit from:

- Knowing why we want change
- Good indicators of success
- True expectations
- Learning how to change eating habits, which is a process, not a timeline
- Overcoming resistance to changing eating habits
- Simple, usable tools that teach awareness and self-experimentation to find what works for you
- Repetition of what works, which creates new habits that work

Ending up with a body you don't recognize as the true *you* took years. Returning your body to the true you, and maintaining it, requires a lifetime of change. Reliable success indicators keep you working in the right direction. You change and improve by staying focused—that is, thinking about what you eat at every meal, with every snack, for the rest of your life. Positive change begins with connecting the dots between how the food you eat affects how you feel and perform.

Do you want change? Why? When you know the *why*, the *how* becomes much easier.

Spend time becoming clear on why you want change. Is it so that you have more energy to play with your kids or grandkids, or to travel, or to return to your favorite sport? When you recapture the true you, you are more ready to give your unique gift to the universe. Your life purpose will blossom.

The One Hour Power Diet is focused thinking that creates change.

Anyone who has lost weight and began a life of feeling good did it by changing eating habits…for a lifetime.

Awareness is the key to all change.

Maybe we should start listening to our body and measure food energy, not by the inaccurate calorie method, but by how much energy we have one hour after eating.

Our bodies talk to us. It's time we start listening. *The One Hour Power Diet* gives you some tools to learn how.

Start with this:

Ask why you are eating just before you eat: for nutrients, for pleasure, or because of an unmet need like lack of love or lack of fulfillment→ Then 1hr power: one hour after eating, rate how much energy and mental clarity you have, as well as how your body feels in general→Visualize the type of food you ate and serving size: one serving=one palm size meal, two servings=two palms, three=three. Start realizing that certain foods and how much you eat make you feel good and certain foods and volumes make you feel bad. Track both the feel-bad choices and the feel-good choices.

Again:

- Answer why you are eating before you eat
- Check in with yourself one hour after eating—that's the One-Hour Power check-in
- Note the serving size of what you ate, your palm as a guide, and log the type of food you ate
- Rate how you feel
- Develop your own personal feel-good/feel-bad database
- Choose feel-good most of the time

Repeating what works over time creates a new habit.

This book is loaded with perspectives that create awareness and keep you focused and moving in the right direction, and tools that build repetition.

You'll find information about a revolutionary tool and how to get it for free—a unique phone app that helps you develop your personal feel-good food-awareness database.

Remember: the ultimate measure of success is feeling like the *real you* … not the *you* carrying extra pounds, too tired and foggy-headed to live your passions.

One hour per meal will give you power.

Overcoming Weight-Loss "Infobesity"

CHAPTER 1

We have been brainwashed.

Do you wonder why we keep doing the same things with the same results—that don't work—be it war for peace or the new magical diet for weight loss?

Are you open to the possibility that our thoughts have been conditioned, and in a sense brainwashed into believing that something we've tried before will work this time? Same story, same results, over and over. The problem with our food choices is we have been conditioned through marketing and hype and weak science to believe we should eat in a certain way.

It's your time to change. Now is the time to find lasting solutions, not short-term results. Now is the time to do something different. Now is the time to give up our loyalty to these conditioned thoughts.

This chapter helps you re-examine the dogma that keeps you going down a path that doesn't work and embark on a path of success. Success through awareness.

If you want to change, you must change your thoughts. Think of this chapter as the beginning of a journey. A journey that may change the way you think about food and food choices.

So we will *look at what we are currently doing*, and the science behind what we do, and take a closer look at expert advice. Usable, reliable, *expert* advice comes from experience, not from weak science. So we'll take a bit of a detour in "Chapter 2: Experience Is the Foundation of Expertise" and examine my experience so you develop trust in my guidance, trust to believe in a perspective that's a bit different. Then maybe you will trust me to show you what to pay attention to, what things mean, how things work, how to advance, and how you might find the real you, not the you with a body overweight and out of balance.

In beginning this journey, understand that we have become *food information-oholics*, because we're starving for information that will work.

We commonly hear someone talk about the amount of calories in this or that, the number of fat grams in this or that, the number of sugar grams in this or that, and so on.

The bad news is most of the information we accept as dogma is scientifically inaccurate and often misleads us into believing if we do X then Y will happen. This creates false expectations.

False expectations make us want to quit.

It's better to find what works and not quit.

Almost every day we hear, "This study proves X." Later, we hear, "This study proves the opposite of X." We feel confused and confusion makes choosing a path and sticking to it difficult or impossible. The only way you will have long-term success is to stick to a path that works for you.

Often these studies claim results in the name of science, and that's where the confusion begins. What is science?

Science is a process of experimentation where we discover reliable rules to predict an outcome. It requires a trial-and-error approach and proves something only if the experiment can be repeated with the same results. So if some method of weight loss really works for most people, then the experiment should be able to be repeated with similar results by some other group.

So if X method of non-surgical weight loss is a lasting solution, there should be a study where several hundred or thousand have been enrolled in the study, and some reasonable percentage of those enrolled went through the process and lost 50% of their excess weight and were able to keep it off for at least five years. Then the method should be repeated to see if the results are reproducible. Guess what? No such study exists. All those claims and no study can do this. Isn't that amazing!?

Here's an example of statistical wizardry: because a certain foot size may correlate with a better understanding of math doesn't mean a bigger foot size causes a better understanding of math. It's because a sophomore in high school has a bigger foot size than a six-year-old and a sophomore is old enough to understand math better.

Correlation does not prove causation.

So beware when some expert says, "The science shows this and the science shows that" and uses statistical wizardry. Beware of terms like *confirms* or *conclusively shows*. These studies may show a correlation, but that doesn't prove *cause*. "Experts" should use phrasing like "suggests or highly suggests." Also beware of the belief that before-and-after pictures mean some process would work for you. The pictures prove short-term results for the person in the picture.

The purpose of this book is to elevate your awareness about what it means to eat and feel better. This book will help you shift away from taking any food information as dogma toward your own personal trial-and-error approach to finding food and ways to eat that help you feel better.

So let's run through some examples of dogma that's misleading and based on weak science by looking at what we are currently doing.

Look at what we're doing:
- We measure food energy with calories
- We measure the amount of protein, fat, and carbohydrates we eat by how much they weigh, in grams
- We measure obesity with the Body Mass Index (BMI)
- We measure our nutrient intake by looking at food labels
- We measure success by the number of pounds lost on the bathroom scale and by how fast we lose those pounds

Look at the science:
Calories are measured by burning food in a calibrated box with a flame. When the food burns, it releases heat. The amount of heat released that can raise one gram of water one degree centigrade is a calorie. Our body does not burn food…it digests food. Millions of complex things happen when we digest food, and no physiologic process in our body resembles burning food with a flame. Burning grease on a fire will feel very hot. Burning bark, which is a carbohydrate, or a piece of meat, will feel less hot. Fat has approximately nine calories per gram, and carbohydrates and proteins approximately four calories per gram. These numbers are based on how hot they burn, not how the body uses the nutrients for energy or energy storage. While measuring heat is a way to measure energy in physical science, it is not how our body

handles food and uses energy. The concept is not based on physiology and is fundamentally flawed.

The way to measure food energy is to ask yourself how much energy you have after eating. Duh! Sometimes, the right answer is right in front of us.

Here's another example: Just because fat has more than twice the calories as protein, it does not mean that it makes you twice as fat. Yet, that's what we have been conditioned to believe.

The physical weight (in grams) of a protein or a carbohydrate or a fat has weak scientific correlation with how much of that nutrient we need to function properly or what percentage of our diet should contain that nutrient. You could grind up horse hooves, a protein, and weigh it to produce a number to list as grams of protein. That number tells you nothing about how well your body would utilize that protein. So when a product says it has eight grams of protein, it's telling you how much it weighs and little else.

The digestive process has evolved over millions of years. Millions of functions contribute to how a food nutrient is digested and used. How well our body utilizes a food depends on how well it is digested and absorbed, not by how much it weighs. So in my opinion, how much a nutrient weighs has very little to do with how well our body will utilize it.

We measure obesity with the BMI, a numerical measurement of how much you weigh divided by how tall you are, with a correction factor for pounds and inches. BMI doesn't account for differences in lean body mass, like bone or muscle. You can be lean and have lots of muscle and bone, and your BMI will be high. Everybody in the nutritional sciences knows that BMI is inaccurate. Yet, it's how we measure obesity.

You can look at someone and tell if that person is obese. What makes measuring calories, grams of nutrients, and BMI so wrong is they are the numbers used in almost all the scientific studies. The excuse for using them, despite knowing their pitfalls, is the acknowledgement that nothing better to use is available. When it comes to scientific studies, inputting flawed numbers delivers flawed results. Garbage in = garbage out.

We measure the nutrients in our food by reading food labels. The majority of food labels are created with food-analysis techniques. Most big food manufacturers test their foods before, during, and after manufacturing to create the nutrient information for their labels. However, the FDA allows a 20% deviation of error—meaning the FDA allows manufacturers and packagers a surprisingly wide latitude in food ingredient "truth." The ingredient information can be off by 20% in either direction and still be in compliance. For instance, if the label says that a food contains 300 calories, it may actually contain anywhere from 240 to 360 calories. The same margin of error goes for other nutrients as well, which isn't very safe for diabetic carb counters, or people with high blood pressure who are watching sodium intake, or mothers looking to boost the iron content of their infants' diets. The FDA has never established a random label-auditing process, and compliance with the law is self-enforced by food manufacturers. This leaves lots of room for inaccuracy due to variation.

The biggest value of food labels is that the information on them gets us thinking about what we're about to eat. That's important. Just realize your body will respond differently to different saturated fats, to different proteins, and to different carbohydrates. Another big problem with food labels is all ingredients don't have to be listed—only the most prevalent. Some minor ingredients may be affecting us badly.

We measure success by the number of pounds lost on the bathroom scale and by how fast we lost those pounds. We have heard all the statement "lose seven pounds in seven days."

Have you been told to weigh yourself first thing in the morning? You know why? It's because you are dehydrated from seven to ten hours of sleep without taking in liquids. In contrast, if you weigh after a binge of high-salt-content food, you will have gained a few pounds. This is water weight. When we weigh, we want to know pounds of fat lost. Long-term and as a trend, this kind of weighing is accurate within five pounds. Short-term, it is very inaccurate. The best way to see the gradual progress from your diet changes is to monitor changes in clothes size. Why? Because it is a simple measure of volume. Volume changes most reflect changes in fat and muscle. It's easy to find many ways to lose water weight quickly, and that's what quick weight loss accomplishes. There is some value though. Excess water weight feels the worst of all excess weight.

If you have been working hard on changing your eating habits with some diet change and you get on the bathroom scale and do not see the results you were expecting, then you will have inner voices saying, "This is not working." Then you will want to quit. Instead, monitor changes in your clothes. Your clothes size will progressively change and is a true indicator of success.

We also tend to believe any expert that uses the word "science" or scientific-sounding words, like grehlin. Grehlin is one of hundreds, if not thousands, of obesity-related peptides. They all work in concert with each other. So when some expert says, "Do this because it affects grehlin levels," they're trying to sound like an expert but not really sharing useful information and possibly know very little about obesity-related peptides. Have you ever heard that you need to eat certain foods to make your body more alkaline? Just using the word alkaline makes the experts sound like they know what they're talking about. But our body physiology maintains a very tight pH balance, primarily with the kidneys and respiration rapidly compensating for any changes. Food doesn't shift that pH balance. If we get too acid or too alkaline, our body rapidly corrects it to maintain balance. And if we do have sustained shifts in more alkalinity, we die.

It may be that eating "alkalizing foods" makes us feel better, and if they do, we should eat them, but it's not because they change the body's pH. So be careful of expert advice. Be an open skeptic and do your homework. Become your own nutrition expert.

False information creates false expectations, and false expectations make us want to quit. If you are looking for lasting solutions and not short term results, then it's time to give up these poor indicators of success and look for quality indicators of progress towards success. The best monitor that you are on a path to success is to begin paying attention to how your daily eating habits are changing, month by month and hopefully year by year. Those habits have been around for a long time and do not change overnight. Monitor your clothes size changing. Monitor your energy, mental clarity, and how your body feels changing. Do this by checking in one hour after eating. Remember the food and food volume and rate how you feel. Rate your energy, mental clarity, and how your body feels. Choose feel-good food.

One Hour Power—one hour can change your life,
and it takes only minutes.

This book features a chapter on "Tools for Success—Changing Your Eating Habits, Changing Your Life" (Chapter 9). You may want to skip ahead and read that chapter to get the core of suggestions. And we have the mini-book *Tools for Success* available so you can easily carry it with you and read it many times. Go to www.changeyoureating.com to get your copy.

The next chapter is my story, so that you can trust my advice. With trust, the "Tools for Success" chapter can be more meaningful and deliver the power of weight loss and energy gain.

CHAPTER 2

Experience Is the Foundation of Expertise

E xpertise comes from experience. Experts give advice. Following that advice requires work. Work takes energy. So maybe, before you take action and use your precious energy on a new journey of change, you should know the experts' story.

While reading this book, you will have moments where those inner voices say, "I have never heard that before." The following stories are where that perspective comes from. Not because I am an M.D., but because of the more than three decades of my *unique experiences as an M.D.*

I think I have the best job on the planet. I will share with you various stories and experiences, and each story will share a take-away message.

In the fall of 1988, I was lying in bed with my wife in a deep sleep. Around midnight I received a call that a 12-year-old boy had been shot with a .22 rifle in the chest and had no vital signs. I was the

Chief Resident and was required to attend all major life-threatening traumas. I really didn't want to get out of bed to go pronounce a 12-year-old dead…but was he? So within a few minutes I *showed up* at the ER just as the boy arrived. I was in my *zone* instantly. I asked if anyone knew how long the boy had no pulse. It was a moment where time slowed and awareness peaked. I could see every face all at once and knew no one knew. I knew every second mattered. I saw a bag of clean laundry. I grabbed the laundry bag and used it to prop the boy on his side as I asked the head nurse for a scalpel blade. No handle, just the blade, no sterile drapes, and with my bare hands I took the blade and opened the boy's chest. I pushed his lungs out of the way, opened the pericardium and saw a heart with a hole in the ventricle and no blood in the heart. He was still warm, so I knew I had a shot at getting him back. I took a pair of scissors and cut off the corner of the left atrium and took unsterile IV tubing and put it in the atrium and sutured it in place. Within a minute or two we were able to get several units of blood pumped in. Then I started massaging the heart. Then my heart exploded with exhilaration as I saw that boy's heart come to life and start beating. After that, we took the time to put on sterile gloves and some drapes and splash everything with betadine and sutured the holes. From the moment I walked into the ER to this moment was less than five minutes. My eyes became watery with joy as I saw his pupils react to light. He was going to be OK! I knew for that boy, at that moment, no one else could have done what I did. I was in my zone. And it mattered.

I became very good at trauma, one step at a time. Baby steps of experience.

I will never forget my first night as the general surgery resident. I had the night duty. After making rounds, I went to the call room to lie down and get some sleep. My heart was beating so hard everything seemed to vibrate. I could imagine a "code blue" or some other immediate emergency happening where I would get the first call and be expected to show up first and do something. I didn't know if I could do it.

I was scared, and also very alive. So I got up and went to visit the Intensive Care Unit nurses. Just talking to them calmed me down. The truth was they knew a lot more about running an effective code than I did. Why? Because of the experience of being present and participating in many codes. They were experts because of experience. And if there was a code, they would have my back and the patient would get the care they needed.

I was lucky. I started my residency in general surgery with an excellent team. The fourth-year resident was Mike Sarap. Mike taught me a lot. Mike taught me how to show up and get it done. He taught me how to take it one step at a time. If, during rounds or any activity, there was a code blue, we would stop everything and run full throttle to the code. At first I thought, that's the internal medicine guy's job, let's do the surgery stuff. Mike 100% believed we could do it better. And after all, "this could be your grandmother." "It matters." At first it seemed like there were too many things happening at once and that made it difficult to know what to do. I learned from Mike to find one thing to do, and do that. After that, find one thing to do, and do that. Before long I was able to do it all and do it fast. So as a young resident, when facing a life-threatening trauma, I learned to walk in with confidence and find one thing to do at a time. After three to four years of this step-by-step learning, it was my time to be "the guy." The gunshot boy survived because I knew every second mattered and I had the experience. I went from a scared first-year resident to peak performance.

Your Take-Away
- **You must show up and do the work. Doing the work really does matter.**

- **Experts come from experience. Experience happens one step at a time. Learn from my experience—it's time to start your self-experiment and find the foods that work best for you.**

So how the heck did a trauma surgeon become an eating advice expert? Read on. I think you will find it interesting and you will better understand why my perspective sounds a bit different, or at least is something you have not heard presented in this manner. Hopefully these stories will open you up to some methods to try and, through self-experimentation, find what works for you. Your goal is to tap into your personal awareness of how the food you choose to eat affects how you feel and perform each day.

Almost all my life has been leading to this. My dad was the hospital administrator of my uncle's hospital. I begin working there when I was ten. I worked in maintenance for about five years before I moved into hospital work. I started in the x-ray department. My job was to transport patients, but because I paid attention and asked questions, I soon started taking x-rays and was good at it. I found how fast the day went by and found that helping patients felt good.

Later I went to work in the lab. This was back in the day where we would conduct some test like detecting cardiac enzymes for possible heart attack patients, with glass pipettes. It was a real chemistry study done with control samples. If I did the test right, the control sample would have a specific reading. If I did the steps wrong, the control sample reading would be wrong. At that young age, I had some high school chemistry, but this was the real deal. Each lab chemistry that we ran was a control study. All good studies have control samples.

Your Take-Away
- This is one of the big problems in doing nutritional/ eating right research. It's difficult or impossible to find a representative control group and to control all variables. If you can control the variables, you know that doing This causes That.
- Almost all types of research prove some correlation, but it's very difficult to prove causation.

Later I began working in the operating room with my uncle, the surgeon and healer extraordinaire. I decided that was the best job ever and committed to becoming a doctor. I already knew I felt good when helping patients. Now I knew where my talents and passion intersected. At that moment and for the next six years, I followed my uncle around almost every day. I saw his skills in the operating room, but what I learned most was his ability as a healer. He just seemed to know what the patient needed. Sometimes he would just sit there with the patient and tell boyhood stories. I would watch as the patients responded and it was amazing. He knew that sometimes the patient didn't need a pill, shot, or surgery; that person just needed reassurance from a doctor they trusted and who was there for them.

Your Take-Away
- Experts have experience that often comes from great mentors. My uncle was an amazing mentor.
- Look for eating-right advice from experts that have experience and great mentors.
- Look beyond the marketing hype. Use your energy to change wisely.

The real birth of nutrition started with the work of one of my general surgeon predecessors, Dr. Stanley Dudrick. I bet that's something you have never heard before! Who would guess that surgeons trained to take out gall bladders and the like are some of the forefathers of nutritional information.

It began by trying to figure out how to keep tiny premature babies from starving to death. Often they had issues where they could not be adequately fed by mouth, so we had to figure out how to feed them with IV fluids that we call TPN (Total Parenteral Nutrition).

The history of TPN is a story of experimentation using the trial-and-error approach to finding what works. Dr. Dudrick and his team had a relentless passion to find what works and learn from what didn't work. They knew from biochemistry what chemicals the various body pathways needed to function, but they didn't know how much to supply those pathways or how to supply the chemicals so that the body would accept the supply.

At first, they started feeding the premature neonates with concentrated glucose solutions, which would switch the body from breaking down cells for food (catabolism) to building cells for growth (anabolism). But they found this much glucose caused the production of too much carbon dioxide. The only way to get rid of that excess carbon dioxide was to breathe the baby very fast with a ventilator. The problem was that as the baby was doing better, they could not wean them off the ventilator. So they began adding calories using amino acids and, later, fat.

They learned that the body needs more than calories; it needs specific nutrients. They also found that the lack of amino acids caused liver failure, the lack of fat caused scaly skin issues, and the lack of trace elements caused many specific problems like anemia, neurologic problems, skin pustules, movement issues, and more. At first, they would introduce fat by rubbing it on the baby's skin and later figured out how to introduce it in the IV fluids. They would add a new nutrient every few days and observe the response and arrive at the appropriate dosage. Too much was a problem; not enough was a problem. That's when many of the nutrient requirements were established. And today, this experimentation is one of the main reasons pre-mature neonatal mortality has improved.

Most of my career has been involved in high-risk surgery that often involves TPN.

Your Take-Away

- **The trial-and-error approach to nutrition has a proven track record and has been responsible for much of what we know about nutritional requirements. Catabolism, the breaking down of cells, and anabolism, the building of cells, have a delicate balance.**
- **A body in balance doesn't excessively break down tissue for food. So stop starvation diets—they only throw your body further out of balance.**
- **We are still learning what we need. The body needs more than calories; it needs specific nutrients.**

I have been heavily influenced by my extensive experience taking care of neonates and burn patients. My residency program had the only neonatal intensive care unit and burn unit in West Virginia. I ended up on the pediatric surgery rotation where I would make daily rounds in the NICU for 11 months out of the five years of my residency. Very few residents get such an extensive experience. That's where I learned a lot about fluid balance. For those tiny premature babies, every drop of fluid mattered. It was easy to give too much and not enough.

I spent a third of my residency at the hospital with the burn unit. The entire team participated daily in the care of patients who'd burned

60% their bodies—or more. That patient would require about 20 bags of IV fluids in the first 24 hours of the burn to maintain normal blood pressure.

For the neonates, we used five primary parameters: skin turgor, urine specific gravity, body weight, urine output, and changes in the lab value of electrolytes. After the burn patient was stabilized, we would look at blood pressure and hourly urine output, knowing the normal urine output is about 0.5cc per kilogram per hour—or for an average adult, about 50 cc per hour.

Your Take-Away
- **Much of my advice comes from these experiences. For example, in the "Tools for Success" section of this book, the information about the best way to monitor that you are drinking enough liquids (urinating about every three to four hours), came from this experience.**
- **Also, my discussion of using a refractometer to measure your urine specific gravity as a learning experience, as a way to know if you are hydrated or dehydrated, comes from past experience.**

To wind up this *experts have experience* chapter, I would like to share my experience in the area of the gastrointestinal tract. Medical students learn microanatomy in medical school. That's the foundation that allows us to examine a piece of tissue through a microscope and determine if it's normal or abnormal. I spent two months of my residency in the pathology department. I reviewed slides of tissue, ranging from the tongue to the anus. I have also spent the last 30 years performing endoscopy, where I would look from the tongue to the anus with a scope. The gastrointestinal tract became my passion. Though I did surgery on every aspect of the GI tract, I also medically managed issues ranging from irritable bowel syndrome (IBS) to inflammatory bowel disease.

In the early '90s, I became an expert in irritable bowel syndrome. I attended international meetings where the most prominent experts gathered. It taught me a lot about what we didn't know. I listened to the elimination diet expert speak on the difficulty of getting patients to eliminate foods properly and get reliable results. Today, we're better informed about the main culprits of food intolerance, and I will later share tools to find which foods your body does not tolerate. I listened to the researcher who spent his career measuring and correlating bowel gas with symptoms. That taught me about gut sensitivity.

My experience treating patients with IBS taught me the most. It's where I began teaching patients to self-experiment to find what works for them. I would teach patients how to self-train to have better bowel movement habits. Better bowel movement habits fixed much of IBS symptoms. The advice is simple, but came from my experience of treating children with severe functional constipation. In pediatric surgery clinic, we saw about 10 patients with severe constipation each week. We needed to figure out if they had a disease called Hirshsprungs versus what we called functional constipation. Hirshsprungs required surgery and functional constipation required bowel-movement training. The advice teaches awareness of the urge to have a bowel movement. Our bowel wants to move when we get up in the morning and or after a meal. We can prove that by measuring motility. What we learned is some people can feel the increased motility as an urge and some can't. When you can't, that's a problem of awareness, not disease.

I have been suggesting that patients go gluten-free for 25 years. I used to think that gluten sensitivity affected 25% of the population, and then I decided 70% of the population, and now I think 100% of the population. I realize the medical community had it wrong many years ago. We would test for celiac disease, which is uncommon, and if the test was negative, we would not recommend going gluten-free. I decided the test was nearly useless unless someone was anemic and malnourished and experienced bowel movement issues. I found that patients could do a self-test where they would go gluten-free for two weeks and acknowledge how they felt and then do a provocative test by eating something gluten, like pizza, and see how they felt. Patients that have more severe gluten sensitivity report that about 80% of their symptoms resolved within 72 hours.

Your Take-Away
- **The gut and "gut brain" are very complex and still poorly understood. The best way to find what works is by doing self-experimentation and awareness training.**
- **Gut sensitivity is one way our body is talking to us. Developing gut sensitivity awareness of how you feel when your stomach is stretched with food will help you understand that you feel better if you keep that volume small.**
- **Gluten or the way gluten arrives at our gastrointestinal tract is making us sick. Avoid gluten.**

The beauty of a 30-year surgical career is that I can choose where I most prefer to spend my time. Now the majority of my practice is bariatric surgery for weight loss. It's where my skillset and passion has most intersected. Weight-loss surgery is only a tool to help someone change eating habits. If patients don't change their habits, they will regain some or all their weight lost, just like they would with a non-surgical weight-loss diet. If your weight and medical problems qualify you, weight-loss surgery is a very good tool to help you lose the weight and change eating habits.

I am a bit different from many of my colleagues. I do the surgery and then for 12 months, I coach the patients to better eating habits. For 15 years, I have heard patients' struggles and have learned how to better communicate how to get around those struggles and achieve success.

Your Take-Away

- No method of weight loss fits all. Weight-loss surgery may or may not be for you. But you can benefit from learning how to listen to your body and, through awareness and self-experimentation, begin to find what works for you.
- The advice in this book is more about a process. A process that almost everyone, even those with normal body weight, could benefit from. Try the suggestions and see if they work for you. Try advice from experts with experience and see how they work for you.
- The ultimate goal is a body in balance that has energy and mental clarity, and a body that feels good.

CHAPTER 3

You Are the Goal—And You Are the Solution

Think for a minute: What *is* the real you?

In my medical practice, I find many specific reasons my patients decided they need help. They start out by saying, "I just want to be healthier and feel better." As I probe deeper, the real reason comes to life.

What is the real reason you want to learn to eat healthier, lose weight, and achieve a body in balance? It's important to know *why* because then the *how* becomes much easier.

Is it because:

- You are too tired and short of breath to play with your kids?
- Your knees or back hurt?
- You find it difficult to shop for clothes that fit and look good?

- You want to feel confident when your mate wants to be intimate?
- You are tired of food cravings?
- You want to get rid of medicine for hypertension, diabetes, and high cholesterol?
- You don't like the way you look in pictures because you don't feel it represents the real you?
- You want a body that moves better?
- You are tired of being sick?

Do you yearn for a day when:
- You can wear what you want and look good, like the real you?
- You actually look forward to clothes shopping?
- You can do the sports you love with the skills you know you have?
- You know you are no longer a sick person on lots of medicine?
- You can easily cross your legs?
- You can inspire others to eat well?

What activities do you enjoy most, yet make you uncomfortable because of your weight? What represents success to you? What are your goals? Picture them.

Visualization is a powerful force inside our minds. It's the method that our conscious brain uses to communicate with the deeper sections of our mind, the subconscious.

Your subconscious mind is constantly filtering information almost 24 hours a day—(yes even in your sleep!) and using that information to construct what it thinks your life should look like. At an early age your subconscious formed its own set of "rules" about itself, and about "you" in the process.

Your subconscious routinely fits all the information that's swirling around you every day into nice patterns and groups that align with the rules it's made about you over time.

When you try to change the rules, to lose weight for example, your subconscious mind starts to look for a group or pattern to fit this new information into… but in many cases it doesn't exist, or there's some block in place to prevent you from really being open to reaching that goal.

That's where visualization comes in. Remember, it's the conscious brain's way of communicating important information directly to the subconscious. In this case, you want to lose weight, and you need to make your subconscious mind aware of what you want… and WHY you want it.

Awareness is the key to making the change. Becoming fully aware of what you want… why you want it and then using the power of visualization to make it become "true" to your subconscious unlocks the power of your subconscious mind to allow it to start to actually happen in your life.

When you can actually see and feel the new, thinner and more incredibly healthy "you" and you share that with your subconscious by using visualization, you're igniting the spark of truth that can allow you to start to see those positive changes emerging in your life.

Awareness is the key to all change. It starts with knowing why you want change and visualizing what the real you looks and feels like.

So here are some questions to help you start to create a clear mental picture of what you want your future self to become.

- Can you, with full clarity, picture in your mind what you're trying to achieve?

- Do you remember what it feels like to be healthy, fit and carefree?
- What value would you place on having that feeling in your life again right now?
- Be 100% clear on WHY you want to change, what that would look like, what that would feel like… try to see and feel it as if it's happening right now.

When you discover your true "why" then you'll start to uncover the real you.

For some people, especially just starting out, the concept of visualization can be a little tricky.

So I reached out to a friend who has some of the most cutting edge programs available right now to aid in this kind of visualization.

My friend Natalie Ledwell and her team at Mind Movies have developed a very powerful, very simple little tool to take ALL the guesswork out of your visualizations, and she's agreed to do me a favor.

You see a Mind Movie is pretty much exactly what it sounds like, it's a visualization tool that uses a short 3-4 minute movie to help you visualize the goal you want to achieve—in this case weight loss and vibrant health!

All you have to do is watch this specially designed Mind Movie 2 times a day, once when you wake up, and then once just before bed and it starts to imprint on your subconscious the fantastic new and positive patterns of weight loss and fitness that you're trying to achieve.

In just a couple minutes a day, your subconscious mind starts to become reprogrammed with your new goals inside it. This allows you to rapidly start to achieve your goals quicker than you might have thought possible.

So not only did Natalie share some thoughts with me about how powerful visualizations actually are for reaching goals, but she also told me to give you a special free gift—It's a 100% Free Pre-made Mind Movie that's specifically designed for your vibrant health and weight loss goals.

All you need to do to grab your personal copy is go here: www. mindmovies.com/weightloss.

Get your new Mind Movie, start watching it, and see just how powerful these visualizations can actually be!

The most I have weighed is 20 pounds more than I do now and I am in shape. But after the early years of raising my children and being very busy with my medical practice, I woke up one day and found myself out of shape and overweight. I was getting short of breath while putting on my shoes! I did not feel like me—athletic and able to ski the black slopes with moguls, slalom ski aggressively, ride motocross, and hike in high altitude. I didn't like the way I looked in a bathing suit picture following a scuba-diving adventure. It just didn't seem like me.

I started working out with a trainer. I found myself getting more physically fit but still not feeling right. I began eating as I taught my patients and gradually developed solid eating habits. Getting physically fit did not do it. Learning to eat well is what made the most difference. The day that I woke up and said to myself, "it's time to change" was a pivotal moment for me

Now I feel as though I am getting younger. I can do what I could do in my twenties and it is most attributed to learning to eat in a way that allows me to have energy, mental clarity, and a body that feels good. I feel like me. Twenty pounds may not seem like a lot, but for me it was disabling.

If carrying extra weight keeps you from feeling like the real you, it's time to do something about it. Learn to choose food that gives you energy, mental clarity, and a body that feels good. You will be well on your way to success.

Solid eating habits + nutritional awareness = the real you.

It's your time! That's why.

CHAPTER 4

Getting Real About Eating Healthier and Losing Weight

A re you ready to learn the art of making that picture of yourself come alive, of achieving the goal of becoming the real you?

And it *is* an art. The masters don't create masterpieces with every painting. They pay attention to the brushstrokes, the paint combinations and the visual perspectives that work as they practice their art, and eventually a masterpiece emerges. Creating the masterpiece that is the true you is a matter of observing what combinations of food and other elements work, and how they make *you* feel. How you eat is how you feel.

We all have different tastes, and we respond differently to various foods. Most of us tolerate milk, but some don't. Some of us can eat eggs; some can't. The food you should eat is the food that makes you feel like the real you.

The trial-and-error method that I advise allows you to eliminate the methods that experience has proven unsuccessful. Quick weight-loss methods ask that you do something that is not sustainable. If you can't keep doing something long-term, it won't work long-term.

Getting real about what we should eat

Here's a primary example of bad/misunderstood science: among all the nutrition advice we've taken as "fact" is the USDA food pyramid. It was useful because it made us think about the food we eat. Yet, it emphasized grains—I'm sure you remember all the health claims about eating wheat bread. Yet, most of those grains contain gluten, which is making us sick and probably is leading us to gain weight, as well. If we were using the trial-and-error method to go gluten-free and see how we feel during that trial, we would have realized the true impact many years ago. Most people that go completely gluten-free can feel a difference in 72 hours. Usually they feel 70-80% better in many ways. Try this approach and see if you feel better.

I suggest a different pyramid. A pyramid to show us how to learn to eat better.

I'll discuss these items in greater detail throughout this book, but let me touch on some critical first actions to take toward changing your eating habits and changing your life.

Put your goals in perspective.

Don't think of the process of becoming healthier, feeling better, and losing weight as

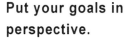

Be you!

Become a nutrition expert

Stay focused on your eating habits

Overcome the resistance to change

Identify the tools that will help you reach your goals

Decide to change your eating habits permanently

a regimented diet. That sounds like work. And though work is involved, picture the process instead as a set of tools that enrich your confidence in yourself, and that rely on yourself and your strengths. That's not work—that's an enjoyable system for rediscovering what makes you more energetic, healthier, and happier.

Decide to change.

Deciding that you want to permanently change your eating habits is the most difficult challenge of all. When you make that decision, the game changes. You will quit looking for quick weight-loss methods and start learning new eating habits that make you feel good and start living in the body of the real you.

Overcome the natural resistance to change.

Most of the tools I share employ simple *doable* mental tricks. I didn't say *easy*. Using these tools will challenge you, but once you learn to overcome that *resistance* to change using the tools, you will invent some that work best for you. When working to get healthier and lose weight, think more in terms of the process than the method.

Concentrate.

Staying focused on your eating habits is a primary secret to long-term weight-loss success. The day you quit having a self-to-self conversation about what and why you're eating the way you do is the day you're in trouble.

No matter whether you read this book or whether you adopt some other plan or method, if you think about your plan and about eating every day, your likelihood of success is very high. Staying focused is easy when you decide to give it the importance that it deserves. Again, concentrating on a clear image of what it's like to live without those extra pounds will motivate you and sustain you.

Learn what works best for you.

Learning what and how much to eat is critical to long-term success. And that's the core of *The One Hour Power Diet* method. Let's dive into the details in our next chapter.

Your Food, Your Life— Step by Step

CHAPTER 5

H ave you heard of the Twinkie, celery, and bean diet? Did you know that you can lose 30 pounds by limiting yourself to these products?

It's true—for what it's worth, anyway. In an experiment, Dr. Mark Haub, who teaches nutrition at Kansas State University, lost 30 pounds after eight weeks eating Twinkies or other snack foods every three hours, along with vegetables, primarily green beans and celery.

This story demonstrates that almost all diets can point to someone who lost weight on their diet plan. However, no diet plan can show good five-year results unless it demonstrates that the dieters have changed their eating habits in a *sustainable* way.

Could you eat Twinkies, celery and green beans for the rest of your life? Is that diet sustainable? Are any of the fad diets that concentrate on a single set of foods or ingredients sustainable? And in fact, Dr. Haub doesn't recommend duplicating his eight-week experiment, in part because the impact of future health can't be measured. But even more important is that fad diets can throw your body further out of balance. Your goal is to achieve balance, not upset it.

In contrast, *The One Hour Power Diet* method helps you change your eating habits permanently. The method is simple and doable, but following it isn't easy.

The problem is that changing habits is difficult. Unfortunately, making those changes is the only way to achieve lasting results. So how do you do it?

Your eating habits won't change overnight. *The One Hour Power Diet* program takes time and self-experimentation. But here's the reward, what will keep you going—each day that you eat well, you will feel better, and each day that you don't, you will feel worse. Awareness of how you feel will inspire permanent change over time.

The One Hour Power Diet method is a feel-good program, and it all comes down to eating in a way that makes you bursting with energy, full of mental clarity, and not being dragged down by that feeling of over-fullness. No expert can tell you what to eat. *You* know what to eat. You could just use more awareness. *Listen to how your body responds.* This is the core of *The One Hour Power Diet* program.

As you use *The One Hour Power Diet* program, you'll discover that the tools for weight loss are already in front of you. Here's how to build that awareness and regain the real you, step by step. I'll explore a number of specific tips for achieving and maintaining your success throughout this book, but the advice boils down to one central principle: learn to understand how food affects you.

You're the only one that can judge how you feel, and what makes you feel better, and what makes you feel worse. Scientists have spent tremendous effort trying to measure energy production in relationship to food, when the way to measure how much energy you get from eating is simply asking yourself how you feel and then measuring it on your personal scale.

When you become aware of how different your body feels when you eat various foods and become aware of the way you eat food, changing old eating habits to new eating habits becomes much easier. In general terms, the food that you should eat is the food and food volume that makes you feel good one hour after eating and the next morning when you awaken.

Any method that helps you change your eating habits in a way that is sustainable and makes you feel good is a winner. The others are a waste of time.

Are you tired of wasting your time? Are you ready for real change?

The One Hour Power Diet: step-by-step actions

Take these actions in committing to weight loss—and succeeding!

Action 1:   Decide that you want permanent change

Action 2:   Start by "detoxing" for two weeks

Action 3:   Follow some basic eating rules

Action 4:   Learn to self-experiment to find what works for you

Action 5:   Discover and learn the reward of changing your eating habits

Action 6:   Ignore poor indicators of success and pay attention to good indicators

Action 7:   Use tools to help you get the job done and become the real you

To launch and sustain *The One Hour Power Diet*, follow this step-by-step, day-by-day flow of actions:

Day 1

Wake up early and center your thoughts for a moment. Close your eyes and focus on your breathing. Inhale through your nose. Feel the air go into your nostrils and deep into your pelvis. Exhale through your mouth—blow the air out as if it was traveling up your spine and out the top of your head. Perform this exercise for three minutes.

Then spend another three minutes asking your soul why you wish to lose weight or change. Maybe it's because you know that carrying those extra pounds is making it hard to be the dad or mom or grandparent you know you are. Maybe your children or your spouse can't wrap their arms around you in a big hug. Maybe you can't participate in the sports that you love. Maybe you feel grumpy most of the time and know that that disposition isn't you. Visualize the You that you know you are—and will be—without those extra pounds.

Write down three reasons you want to change. Attach a visual image to each. Recall my earlier advice: the image might be a mental picture, or it might be a physical one of the earlier you, or of someone you'd like to resemble, or maybe even an activity or a sport you'd like to enjoy again with family and friends.

Perform this simple exercise daily. It takes only six minutes. Spend three minutes centering your thoughts and spend three minutes becoming clear on why you wish to change. Do you have six minutes to change your life?

Also on this day, begin to change your food environment. It's difficult to change eating habits in an environment that enabled, promoted, and sustained the poor eating habits. It's difficult to eat the less-than-optimal foods if they're not there in the first place.

No snack food = no snacking.

Empty your house, car, and workspace of all but essential food. This is by far one of the best tools to avoid snacking. Keep only whole foods and lean meats around for planned eating.

Day 1 to Day 14

Now "detox" for one or two weeks. Whatever and however you're eating must change. That's what detoxing is all about—getting away from your usual eating and drinking habits and what I like to think of as a *taste bud* reset. You'll feel some withdrawal so remember how uncomfortable these withdrawal symptoms feel and write them down. You'll likely need to recall these feelings later.

You will detox by making smoothies in a blender. During this stage, you will basically be on a liquid diet. The magic comes from adding refined coconut oil to the mix. Generally 15-30cc, which is a half or full shot glass. The oil will keep you full and satisfied for three to four hours. If you are feeling too full, decrease the amount of oil. If you require more fullness, add more oil. The goal is to create a high-fiber nutrient-rich drink mixed with the satisfying coconut oil. You can order Nature's Way coconut oil from Amazon.com. If coconut oil is not immediately available and you want to get started, substitute olive oil.

You can also make you own health bar and add this along with the smoothies. Get a combination of nuts, dried fruit, coconut chips, and seeds and blend them together in a blender or buy our "One Hour Power Bar." In my opinion most of the commercially available bars are junk. They contain artificial sweeteners, artificial flavors, refined foods, and chemicals you can't pronounce. Our "One Hour Power Bar" is all organic, gluten free, GMO free, whole real foods, and delicious. You can also buy our version of a powdered green drink to make smoothies. I have tried several and found this to be the most palatable and with the best ingredients. Visit www.changeyoureating. com to order.

In making smoothies, use water, almond milk, coconut milk, or goat milk. Goat milk is not the same as cow milk. In my opinion, goat milk is one of the healthiest drinks on the planet. Drink mostly water for hydration. No soft drinks, no sweet tea, no alcohol, no packaged food, and no candy. No packaged food, no candy.

You're basically detoxing from table sugar, table salt, food additives, artificial sweeteners, gluten, and dairy products. You're eating in a way that will be different. You're not sitting down for meals or grabbing food through a fast-food drive-through. You will lose weight, particularly if you choose to do this for as long as one month. However, I don't recommend continuing this detox regimen longer than one month at a time.

In fact, the "smoothie regimen" is primarily for detoxing or for a taste bud reset. Once you begin working to change your daily eating habits, liquefying your food intake will actually work against natural digestion and absorption of nutrients, thereby reducing the value of the foods you eat; I'll explain why in greater detail in Chapter 9: Tools for Success—Changing Your Eating Habits, Changing Your Life.

After the detox, it's time to learn eating habits that you can maintain year after year. Yes, you'll occasionally revert to old eating habits. If this reversion lasts for more than a few days, you may need to detox again. If you're in danger of slipping back to old habits, recall the uncomfortable withdrawal symptoms you experienced before. You wrote those symptoms down: revisit them. Remember them. Visualize them. Stop those old habits before they re-establish themselves.

Here is a basic farm-to-table recipe for a green smoothie:

½ lemon

3 celery stalks

A handful of spinach, kale, or chard or a combination of each.

1 small whole apple

1 cucumber

A few pinches of ginger

Add water to dilute to your taste

Mix and match the food ingredients that you like from the produce section of your grocery store. Taking time to find what ingredients you like and which ones make you feel the best is the beginning of becoming your own nutrition expert. Remember to become aware of the possible detoxing withdrawal symptoms: headaches, severe cravings, irritability, and more. Any time you see a pattern of bad eating behavior developing, remind yourself that you will need to detox, and when you do, those withdrawal symptoms will once again haunt you.

Remember that changing your eating habits and changing your life is a process, not a timeline. Old habits do not disappear overnight. It takes finding what works for you and then repetitively coming back to what works. Over time, a new habit is formed. If *it's your time* to change, then start the process and do the work.

Day 14 to Day 28

While en route someplace, stop at a grocery store with the intention that you will be in and out in 10 minutes. In the deli section, buy lean cooked meats—for instance, one package of sliced turkey breast. If you wish, buy cheese (high-quality hand-made cheese, not factory-made). In the produce section, select ten items to your taste, such as nuts, spinach, celery, carrots, avocados, cherry tomatoes, bell peppers, apples, oranges, bananas, or any of the other fruits, vegetables, and other items available in that section.

Place what you've purchased in a brown paper bag or your own personal bag—it should be about half full. Carry that half sack of food with you at all times. Every three to four hours, eat something from the bag. Every two to three days, run into the grocery store and restock your bag.

Do this for ten days to two weeks so that you get an idea how it feels to eat clean. You will also recognize how easy such a habit is to achieve and sustain. Many of your daily chores disappear, because those chores are related to eating. For instance, going to a fast food restaurant seems simple and quick, yet the effort of driving to the restaurant, standing in line, placing your order, paying, returning home, unwrapping the food, eating, and then discarding the wrapping takes more effort than running into a grocery store every two days for ten minutes with your brown paper bag in hand. You'll also find that by going to the store every two days, the food you eat is fresh and tastier than anything you could get at a fast food restaurant or many other restaurants.

As you perform your six-minute morning routine of deep breathing and centering your thoughts, ask yourself how you feel. Do you have mental clarity? Do you feel energetic? How does your body feel? Write your feelings down.

Day 28 to 35

Now return to your normal eating habits. Eat fast food, eat salty food, eat sugary food, drink alcohol, eat dairy, and eat gluten-containing food. One hour after you eat, note how your body responded to that particular group of food and/or drink. It's important to conduct these provocative tests so that you become aware that your eating habits are making you feel bad. Checking in one hour after eating can change your life.

It takes roughly an hour for the body to signal its reaction to food, and therefore for you to know whether you ate enough or you overate or whether you have energy or whether you feel like hitting the couch.

You might feel brief satisfaction from some foods, such as the taste of chocolate, within five minutes. However, it takes at least an hour after eating for you to become fully aware of how the food actually made you feel. Take notes one hour after eating.

With that timing in mind, take this approach:

- Log how you feel one hour after eating
- Log the specific foods you eat (red meat, diary, breads, nuts, eggs, etc.)
- Log the source of food (fast food, restaurant, home-cooked)
- Log the portion size of each food
- Log the type of preparation (fried, steamed, raw, etc.)

As you log, ask yourself these questions: *Do you have energy or feel like hitting the couch? Do you have mental clarity or feel foggy? Does your body move freely or sluggishly?* You'll measure in general terms the amount you ate and in general terms the kind of food you ate. The information you provide will create your own personal database, and over time, you'll be able to check your data and see how your eating behavior makes you feel—and which foods and behavior make you feel good and which make you feel like crap.

Then, each morning as you work on breathing and centering your thoughts, ask yourself how you feel, as you did in stage 2. Talk to yourself—and cheer yourself on. Ask yourself these important questions:

- How did you do yesterday? Be honest, but don't beat yourself up if you didn't do as well as you had hoped.
- How do you feel now? Do you have mental clarity? Do you feel energetic? How does your body feel?
- How did you feel one hour after eating?

- Why did you eat what you ate? (We'll explore the possible answers to that question, and the impact of those answers, in Chapter 6: Committing to Changing Your Habits—Are You Ready.)
- Why do you want to lose weight? Remind yourself after each meal.

The day you quit having the conversation about why you're eating and why you want to lose weight and eat healthy is the day you're in trouble.

These questions and their answers are very important. They bring awareness to how your eating habits affect how you feel. Awareness is the key to all change, and changing your eating habits can change your life.

From day 35 to eternity

Continue logging, evaluating, and adjusting your eating habits based on what you discover.

But also realize that sometimes you'll need to backtrack and "reboot" the *One Hour Power Diet* program process. We rarely learn something at first pass. You may have to revisit this pattern several times, because we as humans always run the risk of falling back into old habits. Recognize and admit to yourself how those old habits drained you, constricted you, and sickened you. Detox for another two weeks while feeling those old uncomfortable withdrawal symptoms, and then start eating clean again.

Some experts say it takes 21 days to develop a habit. This takes longer than 21 days. I like to think in terms of chipping away at success. I hope your eating habits continue to improve for the rest of your life. And they will as you learn better awareness and techniques that work for you. This will work as long as you have a clear image of what you are trying to achieve and keep the conversation active about what you are eating and why.

We'll learn more about how to change habits more successfully, and less painfully, in "Chapter 5: Changing Eating Habits Made Easier."

To maximize the benefits of *The One Hour Power Diet* program, follow these approaches.

Experiment with what you eat.

Sample foods you haven't eaten before. Try beets, cabbage, olives, cucumber, celery, parsley, chard, melons, goat cheese, various nuts, kale, mangos, chickpeas, lentils, quinoa, hummus, bean salad, sushi, Cajun red beans, and on and on and on—so many exciting, available foods could energize you and help you break previous habits.

Don't think that experimentation necessarily means exotic, ethnic, or international. Perhaps you grew up in a household that never ate broccoli because one of your parents didn't like it or just never happened to buy it—you might very well fall in love with broccoli or Brussels sprouts or asparagus or peas, but you don't know because of your past. And tastes change. Maybe you didn't like mushrooms as a child and have never eaten them since. These days, you might find that you now actually like them. Or you might like a specific type of mushroom you've never sampled because it just wasn't available back when, but is in your grocery now—and this increased variety can be found in so many varieties of fruits, vegetables, and other foods that are available in the local markets these days.

Break from old habits with new foods. Try them, and log how you feel an hour and a day after eating them. You may very well discover foods that surprise you, empower you, and bring new enjoyment to eating and to changing your eating habits. And you just might find comfort in foods outside of your typical "comfort zone."

Follow basic eating rules and success habits.

The basic eating rules and guidelines are detailed in Chapter 7: Changing Eating Habits Made Easier.

Briefly, these guidelines are:

- Learn what fullness feels like—you have eaten enough long before you feel like it.
- Get comfortable wasting food—for example, always leave some food on your plate.
- Eat breakfast soon after awakening with some fruit and protein (such as Canadian bacon or eggs).
- Eat every three to four hours. Keep your body in rhythm.
- Avoid unplanned eating. Haphazard eating leads to sloppy eating habits.
- Learn to eat slowly. Allow yourself time to feel fullness.
- Eat a volume of food roughly the size of the palm of your hand and up to the first knuckle.
- Start your meal with protein that should be the size from your thumb to the large thumb skin crease.
- Drink mostly water—but avoid drinking water while you eat (it washes away the nutrients too fast)
- Give up packaged, processed food that is full of additives.
- Limit refined table salt, and use Himalayan or Celtic salt.
- Keep your body moving. Exercise promotes body balance and helps you sleep.

Experiment with various foods and weight-loss advice.

Though many experts are crippled with their own the God Complex, some of what they share may work. But the experts don't truly know if their advice works for *you*.

Therefore, test the suggested technique—whether eating vegetarian, the Paleo diet, the low-carb/high-protein diet, the gluten-free diet, the dairy-free diet, or whatever—and see how it makes you feel one hour after eating and then how it makes you feel the next morning.

Try a variety of techniques and find what works for you.

Though the science behind calories and grams of protein, fat, and carbohydrates is poor, calorie-counting or counting grams of protein, fat, and carbohydrates may work for you. You may realize that paying attention to the amount of fat in a meal correlates directly with how full you feel and how much energy you have. This is another way to build awareness.

Do what works, abandon what does not work.

Ignore poor indicators of success and pay attention to good indicators of success.

The One Hour Power Diet method defines success as achieving a feeling of energy, clarity, enthusiasm, and comfort. Yes, your goal is to lose weight and to become healthier. But measure those goals based on *you*, and not on arbitrary and often misleading indicators.

For instance: the pounds lost per day or per week is a poor indicator of success. The scale shows more about your water balance than it does about pounds of fat lost. Instead, pay attention to how your clothes feel—for example, how your shoes and rings feel. Pay attention to how your body moves—for instance, the ease or difficulty of squatting or crossing your legs. Pay attention to your energy and mental clarity. Mostly, pay attention to how your eating habits are changing.

The problem with poor indicators of success like decreasing the amount of calories consumed or watching the amount of pounds lost on the bathroom scale or exercising and expecting pounds of weight to disappear is that they create false expectations, as I'll detail in Chapter 8: Why You Eat What You Eat. When we expect something to happen and it doesn't happen, we want to quit trying.

If you quit, you won't succeed. Monitor how your body is changing, how your eating habits are changing, and how your life is changing—those are the clear indicators of success.

Employ the power of the *The One Hour Power Diet* app tools available to you.

The phone app asks you to photograph each meal for a week. It also asks you to judge the volume of food you ate using the palm of your hand to compare. One serving is one palm, two servings two palms, three servings three palms. You are asked to acknowledge why you are eating. Are you eating for nutrients, pleasure, or an unmet need? Then one hour after eating, you are asked to rate how full you feel, how much mental clarity you have, how much energy you have, and how your body feels—good or bad. This goes to your personal database. After one week the app will show you the pictures of the food and volumes of food that make you feel good and those that make you feel bad. It will also show how often you are eating for nutrients, pleasure, or an unmet need. This takes just a few minutes. We have tried to make it simple and user-friendly. The purpose is to bring awareness to how your food choices affect how you feel and perform.

Get serious about improved well-being, health, and weight loss.

The One Hour Power Diet method succeeds only if you apply its techniques, principles, and overall attitude with dedication and conviction. You must commit to becoming the real you, which is the crucial first step that I'll discuss in the next chapter.

CHAPTER 6

Committing to Changing Your Habits— Are You Ready?

T he #1 challenge to long-term weight loss and healthy-eating success is committing to a process of change—for the rest of your life. Until you're ready to commit, you're wasting your time and energy.

Ouch! This is a bit heavy for an opening paragraph. But this *is* the deal.

Decide. Then do.

If you truly want to lose weight and become healthier, ask yourself: *Am I ready to commit to long-term change?* This process isn't easy, but it *is* doable. Here's how to take the critical next step of commitment in the most effective way possible.

Start by imagining the power of this situation. Let's say that Bob played football in high school. He was lean and he was good. But after high school, he put on pounds year after year. Then came the day when Bob's best friend Mike died suddenly of a heart attack. As Bob put on his suit for the funeral, he was stunned about how poorly it fit. It was tight, constricting. As he looked in the mirror to see where to adjust the pants and the jacket, he saw his best friend. Mike had been overweight, too.

That's when Bob committed to losing weight—and to saving himself. Bob was shocked into waking up. He suddenly realized he would never again share a beer and those quirky jokes that only he and his friend got, because Mike was gone. Worse yet, he now saw himself going down the same path.

Bob had a strong emotional connection to why he wanted to change. Most of us must dig a little deeper to find that true reason for improving our health and losing weight. It's important to spend some quiet time and discover the *why*.

Discover your emotional connection to why you want to lose weight. Then commit.

Can you visualize eating, drinking, and working out like an athlete? Or do you still picture yourself negatively—for instance, as a slob who falls asleep watching TV and wakes up with potato chips all over your shirt?

You've heard the saying, "It's all in the details." A detailed emotional memory is powerful. Experiencing an emotional memory that connects to why you want to lose weight and eat healthy in detail drives commitment. Problem solved.

Maybe you remember days when you were athletic and remember a powerful athletic moment and re-experience in detail how that moment felt. These days, you find that just trying to play with your kids is difficult because of your excess weight. Remember those powerful moments of the past—whether they're athletic achievements or coming into a party feeling confident or fitting into those skinny jeans or whatever it happens to be. Concentrate on the details.

The more emotional memories you have in your tool bag, the better. Search your memories and find them.

However—and this is very important—don't let the memories defeat you. Don't beat yourself up for gaining that excess weight and for eating habits that made you feel terrible. That's the past—the unimportant past—and you can't reverse it.

To a certain extent, you can *recapture* the past, but even then we're looking forward. Commit to change and regain your glory years for your future.

Model your emotional memories like the person you want to be.

I'll warn you: don't wait to decide to lose weight permanently and to do what's required to make it happen. Life is precious.

We're all unique, with special gifts that only we can give to the universe. Reflect back on my example of not being able to play with your kids because of your weight. What gifts are you denying your children, your family, your friends, your community—as well as yourself?

Are you living a life that enables you to give your gift? Does your body work for you, or do you work for your body? Take control and live life as the real you.

Now let's explore how to take control in more detail.

CHAPTER 7

Changing Eating Habits Made Easier

Now that you're committed to the wonderful goal of losing weight, you must change habits. Taking new approaches to eating is just the start, but it isn't enough. Repeating behavior is much easier than learning new behavior.

Overcoming old habits is difficult. Our brain doesn't like to be told that it can't have something it likes and is used to. It doesn't like overcoming obstacles. Our brain likes to continue doing what it knows. It's all about mental inertia. It's a matter of habit.

Still, although habits are often obstacles, they are also powerful tools for achieving permanent change. Changing habits is all about learning new behavior, and new behaviors require attention, concentration, and repetition. To change behavior, we must focus on changing, find what works, and repeat what works many times.

Here's how to develop that focus.

Attack the natural resistance to change.

When you try to change a habit, you will resist, and every day will present obstacles. Resistance and obstacles are painful. Our brain avoids pain and has many tricks to do so—what we refer to as pain-escape mechanisms. But please understand that though pain is inevitable, suffering is not.

Stressful eating is one pain-escape mechanism. Another is rationalization. We can always come up with a good excuse to not do what's painful. For instance, when you start a workout regimen, you will most likely have moments where you're sitting in your car in the gym parking lot thinking of the many reasons you don't have time to work out today. Our brain is really good at this, so beware.

Suffering results when you resist pain. Get rid of the resistance and the pain lessens.

Pain does not equal suffering.
Pain plus resistance equals suffering.

Remind yourself continually of the "why" of your goal.

To shed the resistance to change and the suffering that it leads to, hold on to your clear emotional memory of what you want, as I discussed in Chapter 2: Getting Real About Eating Healthier and Losing Weight. Answering "Why do you want to lose weight and eat healthy?" does far more than simply helping you commit to weight loss. To overcome the resistance to change, remind yourself of that answer every day, at every meal.

Like rushing water in a clear river, emotional experiences will carry you and exhilarate you.

*Feel the emotional experience of what you're trying to accomplish
and the resistance to doing what's required will fade.*

Don't expect instant results.

To avoid frustration that can demotivate you, understand that developing new habits takes time and repetition.

We've all fallen into the "YoYo" diet trap. It's like a carnival game that's impossible to beat, but it lures us into believing we can win, so we keep playing. We all want that healthier feeling, and we all want the extra weight gone, and yesterday is not soon enough. Fad diets promise fast results. But they don't help us lose the extra pounds and keep them off permanently—and we usually regain it all, plus 10%.

Some say it takes 21 days to change a habit, but I like to think in terms of chipping away and getting better and better.

Think back on my story of Bob and his commitment to lose weight in Chapter 6: Committing to Changing Your Habits—Are You Ready? After Bob committed to shedding pounds, he went to a personal trainer. Bob said, "Jack, I need you to help me lose weight and get fit."

Then Jack heard something he'd never heard from a client. "Jack, I gained 40 pounds over five years. I want you to help me lose 40 pounds over the next five years." One thing we know with certainty is that quick weight-loss methods do not work long term. Changing habits works. Our hypothetical friend Bob understood that—and you, in your real world, must understand that, too. You must have a clear emotional view of where you want to be (the why), and not focus on how long it may take.

Bob asked his trainer to help him lose 40 pounds over the long term—not by the end of next month. Learn to love the journey and have realistic expectations.

If you're aware of how you feel as you change, you will achieve your goal and be rewarded daily by how you feel.

The solution to overweight does not occur overnight.

Review your progress regularly.

That's the core of *The One Hour Power Diet* program. Once you know where you're going, you must frequently review where you are.

I'm not talking about a number on a bathroom scale. That number is a goal, yes, but it's not necessarily an effective intermediate measure in accomplishing your goals. The ultimate goal is *how you feel.* And how you feel is a crucial measure of your progress as you chip away at change. Learn what works using *The One Hour Power Diet* program self-education tool. The best indicator of success is monitoring how your eating habits are changing month after month and hopefully year after year.

Besides, if you make yourself aware of your progress—if you feel it and actually taste it—you'll gain another emotional mental image that helps you shed the natural resistance to change. For instance, when you repeatedly experience eating only a small portion of nutritious food that tastes good, and you feel energy and vitality after eating, you're on a path that will change your life. This is true when it comes to food, but it also works in many other life challenges.

At the end of every day, ask how well you did in accomplishing change, in much the same way that you assess how you feel an hour after you eat.

Once you start thinking about your goals and your progress, you will think about them over and over and begin to change the way you feel. Bottom line: build your awareness—particularly about your successes.

Ask yourself how well you did today
and how you can do better tomorrow.

The model of recalling a "feel-good" experience after some difficult task helps you give up the resistance to performing that task and, over time, you become who you are—a person who feels good, and it shows.

Never beat yourself up.

Our daily activities have a rhythm formed from habits. Disrupting that rhythm provokes resistance to change, and this is certainly true of eating habits. And for a while after you disrupt your eating rhythm, your eating habits may get worse. Or you may rebound. For example, maybe you and your loved ones enjoy eating unhealthy food while watching TV, or eating out on specific nights of the week and ordering big portions of guilty-pleasure food. Disrupting this rhythm will hurt. It's just part of the process.

Acknowledge that you may slip a little and binge. Laugh at it. You know what's happening. Just don't let it happen too often. Continue to rely on the tools for changing. As long as you keep chipping away at changing, you will change.

For quick results, become aware of how you feel as you change, because those feelings arise daily if you're on the right path.

Let your brain do its own workout.

Forgive me a moment while I speak in neurological terms: A specific thought develops a neural pathway to that thought. Neural pathways get stronger and wider the more they're used. In fact, frequently used pathways are coated with a physical sheath that makes them even more energy-efficient. Such functions as walking and chewing are powered by strong neural pathways, to the point that you perform them subconsciously. Like Pavlov's dog, which was conditioned to salivate at the sound of bell, we have triggers that send a thought down the pathway of least resistance, and the pathway of least resistance is old habits.

Resistance is built into change, and you will feel that resistance as you try to change. That's where free will comes into play.

Success is not given to us, no matter how gifted we are. Instead, we create our success by what we think, say and do. That sounds as if it's driven by the conscious mind, but I would like to share the story of how DNA married free will and became successful.

Our thoughts drive our bodies and our actions.

DNA is amazing. It determines all life as we know it—it is our program. We may be programmed to be an athlete or a scientist or an artist. DNA makes RNA and RNA makes proteins. Proteins determine how we feel and act. For example, adrenaline makes us want to fight or flee. Oxytocin makes us want to bond and love. Now, here's the link that is a key to changing our eating habits: RNA records information. Every thought we have ever had is recorded in the RNA in the cells of our body. Neural pathways lead to those thoughts. Certain things trigger the pathway to the recorded RNA thought and then the RNA makes the proteins to make our body want to act in that way.

That's where free will comes into play. We choose our thoughts. And in turn, our thoughts signal RNA which proteins to make. The proteins that RNA makes drive our actions. Therefore, our thoughts drive our actions.

Reframe how you think about eating and dieting.

The words we use to ourselves and others matter. Some words open us up. Some words shut us down. And when it comes to weight loss, the words "eating healthy" shut us down. Eating healthy feels like a chore your parents have been nagging you to do, but you resist. "Sit up straight." "Take out the trash." "Clean your room." "Do your homework." And, of course, "Clean your plate."

Instead, use words to yourself that communicate that the benefit of changing a habit outweighs the pain. That's why I recommend that you think of devoting yourself to nutrient eating appropriately balanced with pleasure eating as the "feel-good" diet. We all want to feel good. Reframe your goals with that in mind. Eating better with just the goal of better health rarely works. Eating better because you know what it feels like to eat well and feel good—now *that* works.

After all, when you swim upstream, you feel the resistance of the water. When you swim downstream, you don't feel resistance—and the power of the water helps you swim far more easily. Upstream is "I gotta work to lose weight." Downstream is "I'm feeling better and I'm on my way to feeling great."

This ties into a psychological concept: neuro-linguistic programming (NLP), which provides a way to change our thoughts rapidly. The words we use to ourselves and others can immediately change our physiology. Take the word *fire*. If, as a child, you became aware of fire as you sat in the arms of your father around a campfire feeling warm and safe, then the word *fire* would produce body chemicals like oxytocin that promote bonding. With that background, making love with your significant other in front of a roaring fire would be an off-the-charts bonding moment. However, if you were badly burned as a child, the word *fire* would trigger your body to produce adrenaline. You would feel fear and want to flee.

NLP teaches the concept of "reframing." If you have a thought that triggers a habit you want to change, reframe it in a way that sends the thought down a different pathway, one where different proteins with different physiology are produced. Reframing means choosing different words or thoughts.

Here's an example of how reframing works on an everyday level. Suppose you're at a great restaurant having the best steak you've ever tasted. After you've eaten about three ounces, your mind tells you to keep eating. Yet, as you've used the principles of *The One Hour Power Diet* program, you've learned that you'll feel better one hour after eating if you stop at that point. So instead of saying to yourself, "You can't eat any more steak because you must lose weight and get healthy," you say, "The only thing that changes if I eat more of that steak is how I will feel one hour after eating, and I want to feel good."

You have reframed the situation by describing it differently. You've already paid for the meal and have already enjoyed the taste, and if you "waste it" by not eating the rest, no one will go hungry. Nothing in the world changes except how you will feel after eating. Either you will have energy to do some activity or you will feel like hitting the couch. This reframe—from a chore to a feel-good—shifts eating behavior dramatically.

Success is measured by what we do, but what we do
is inspired by how we think and what we say.

Take the million-dollar challenge.

If I offer to give you a million dollars to build a spacecraft to fly to Mars, you'll reply, "No thanks." Too hard and too expensive.

If I offer to give you a million dollars to ask the waiter at a restaurant to prepare spinach and chopped grilled chicken as your entrée instead of some fattening, unhealthy food on the menu, most likely you'll say, "Yes. Too easy." If I asked you to eat every three hours, you would say things like "I don't have time" or "My life is too busy." But If I asked you to eat every three hours and told you that if you can do this for a month or even a year, you will get the million dollars, you would say, "Show me the money."

If you plan to follow some eating rule, yet you feel resistance to doing it, ask yourself, "If I would be given a million dollars to do this task, would I find it easy?"

When you feel losing weight and eating healthy is worth more than a million dollars, you have commitment to change.

When feeling resistance to change, ask yourself,
"If I were given a million dollars to do this, would I?"

Build awareness of why you are eating.

Why you're eating and *Why you want to lose weight* are different considerations. Answering "Why are you eating?" helps you change habits.

Let's explore the *why you're eating* in our next chapter.

CHAPTER 8

Why You Eat
What You Eat

A key to losing weight and understanding what foods make us feel good is to acknowledge why we eat.

We eat to replenish nutrients, we eat for pleasure, and we eat in an attempt to compensate for unmet needs like love or fulfillment. These unmet needs are dysfunctional because they hurt us in some way.

The "why" of eating helps with the "how" of weight loss.

Ask these questions every time you eat:

- Are you eating to nourish your body, to satisfy hunger, to regain energy, or maybe to promote health and fitness?
- Are you eating for the tastes that you enjoy and have a passion for, or perhaps as a vehicle for socializing with family and friends that share your life or your interests?

- Are you eating because you feel a little beat up from the day and want some comforting love?

With understanding those reasons, we can adjust how and what we eat. Here's how.

Ask are you eating for nutrients, pleasure, or an unmet need?

Eating to fulfill psychological need: compensating for "what's missing" beyond our dinner plates.

You've very likely heard the phrase *looking for love in all the wrong places?*

To extend the analogy, we often eat for love in the all the wrong places. Often the wrong type and the wrong time. Why is it wrong? Because it does not leave us fulfilled and, often, it hurts us.

Most "comfort food" causes discomfort. We might be satiated somewhat after eating such food, but we feel bad physically. Comfort food often causes health problems, and worse, we don't feel good almost immediately. We feel mentally weak for doing it as well as physiologically.

Eating for love in all the wrong places makes us gain weight, lose energy, experience less clarity of thought, and reduces our ability to move and to be the person your soul is trying to show the universe.

Whether our parents taught us to show love through food or whether it's built into our genes, it really doesn't matter. We must deal with it. It hurts us. It's dysfunctional.

Showing love through food is like a couple that loves each other but beats each other up frequently and hurts each other.

Remember the image of a couple that loves each other but beats each other. Recall that image when you feel like eating for emotional reasons, whether it's from a tough day, or because you are angry, depressed, anxious, stressed, lonely, or jealous.

Dysfunctional means "It does not work." So let's talk about what *does* work.

Learn the "love languages" that fulfill you.

We've all had hectic days. Maybe you've been drained by a frustrating day at work. Maybe you've suffered a personal disappointment. Maybe you've worn yourself out with a day of accomplishments and need to relax from the exertion and the stress. In other words, you feel beat up.

When we feel beat up, we want love. We want to be nurtured. We want comfort. And often, no one shows up to give us what we need when we need it most. Turning to food to satisfy such needs is easy and unfortunately hurts us just like the couple that hurts each other's feelings.

For example, you feel beat up from the day, and on your way home you start craving and decide to stop and buy a big bucket of ice cream. You know that if you go home and turn on the TV, you'll eat most of it. If you pay attention to how your body responds, you'll realize the next morning that you are sluggish or thinking less clearly or something not good. Instead, think of your love language and express it in a way that's good for you. Let me explain.

A key to avoiding dysfunctional eating is learning what Gary Chapman calls the "love languages" (in his book coincidentally called *The Five Love Languages*). Chapman describes the primary languages as 1) touch, 2) words of affirmation, like "I love you" or "You're beautiful," 3) gifts, 4) quality time, and 5) acts of service. One or more of these are the way you primarily wish to receive love.

Say your love language is "quality time" and you love a long warm bath with your favorite music. If you feel beat up from a hectic day, then plan time for that bath. If your love language is expressed in "acts of service," get your car washed. If your love language is gifts, buy something you need and love. Personally, my primary love language is touch, but I also like acts of service. When I feel beat up from a busy day, I get a massage. If, for instance, you're the same and massage is not so available or too expensive, consider buying a foot massager.

Tell your family and friends about your love language directly and diplomatically, so they don't comfort you with food.

For example, material "things" don't do much for me. When someone gives me something bought at some store, I don't necessarily feel love. Instead, I question whether the money was well spent. But if someone made me something, or honored me with an act of service, or if they just gave me a body-melting hug, I would cherish it and feel loved.

Asking for love seems needy and is not usually well embraced by those you might be asking to show you love. Learn your love language(s) and learn to give love to yourself and not rely on others. Love yourself in a healthy, functional, non-hurtful way.

Love is about giving, not receiving.

Learn the love languages of your family and friends—other than food.

Recognize that we are driven to show love through food.

Allow me to share a personal story.

My kids were in their early adolescence when my wife and I divorced. My first reaction was to shower them with love. I found myself constantly wanting to feed them bad food. "Let's get ice cream," "Let's order pizza," "Let's get big greasy hamburgers." We didn't normally do those things, and suddenly I wanted to do them, all the time.

There are a number of problems with such an approach:

- I wasn't giving my kids what they really wanted or needed from their dad.
- I wasn't feeding them properly.
- I wasn't feeding *myself* properly—and showing love through food can undermine your work to get healthy and lose weight as much as showing yourself love through food.

When I realized what was going on, I laughed at myself. Despite my awareness of what was happening, I still wanted to continue showing love through food. I laughed at how powerful this need was showing up. Over and over. But I woke up to what I was doing. I became aware. And awareness is the key to all change.

The emotion of showing love through food was powerful. So I continued to be aware of what I was doing and continued to laugh at myself and gradually change. I decided the language of love that I wanted to show them was quality time. I planned adventurous trips: hiking in the Grand Canyon, rafting, camping under the stars and talking. Instead of being overweight, they now have memories of youthful adventures they'll always cherish.

This is especially important in these days of childhood obesity. Nothing is more obviously dysfunctional than childhood obesity. Adults buy the food or give them money to buy the food. They can't get it without our help. I hear patients frequently say they must keep snacks around the house for their kids or grandkids. We like to reward our children with bad food and say things like, "If you're good, you can have some ice cream before bedtime."

Help your family and friends be healthy, and avoid a "comfort food" atmosphere that will also hurt you.

Remember that comfort food can cause discomfort.
Learn how those fast-food hamburgers or pies or cookies or whatever affect you. Do those foods allow you to feel good or fulfilled, or drag you down? Sometimes junk food equals junk mood.

Remember, eating because of stress is a pain-escape mechanism. Instead, shifting your need for love, respect, and comfort from the dysfunctional to the functional is an art, and you are the artist. Only you can paint the picture that works.

Eating for pleasure: appreciating a passionate life.

Great-tasting food delights us, and that's not a bad thing. Yes, taking too much pleasure in eating is one element that gets people into weight problems in the first place, but we can't ignore the importance of appreciating that particular part of our lives.

Still, we must eat for pleasure judiciously and wisely. Here's how:

Give yourself permission to enjoy pleasure food occasionally.
That means that you can look back over a whole month and know that you did it a small number of times. Pleasure is one of the many spices of life. When the time is right, go for it—just don't do it very often.

How do you know the time is right? When it is neither common nor repetitive, and when it's of high quality. If you're in a restaurant that makes the most amazing chocolate cake and you love chocolate cake, I think you would be crazy not to eat some. It's OK. Just don't buy a whole cake, take it home, and eat a piece every day until it's gone. If you do, you'll feel bad mentally and physically.

Be passionate about food, about life.

> *Our body—and, in my opinion, our planet—*
> *has the amazing ability to tolerate pollution,*
> *provided it is neither common nor repetitive.*

Our body and our planet have the amazingly ability to heal themselves rapidly, particularly if the body or planet is "in balance." What it does not tolerate is daily or sustained pollution. Daily or sustained pollution leaves our body and our planet "out of balance."

It's time to get our body and planet in balance.

Skip the guilt.

How often have you eaten food that simply tastes good and then felt bad for doing it? "Next week I will start eating better." "I went on vacation and gained seven pounds. Now I have to make up for it." Has this pattern repeated itself again and again?

Now, tell the truth: have you ever found that beating yourself up for bad behavior truly succeeds in changing that behavior? Beating yourself up for any behavior wastes energy. It is self-defeating. Don't waste your energy on something that doesn't lead you down a path to fulfillment where you can give your unique gifts to the universe. The universe wants you to succeed.

Energy is like money. Be careful how you spend it.

But now it's time to get totally serious about the dangers of pleasure eating and how you can overcome them.

Don't reward yourself with pleasure food.

Eating as a reward gets a little tricky. Yes, you can eat purely for pleasure when the experience is special. This is not a reward—it's a special life moment. For instance, enjoy yourself when celebrating an anniversary, a new job, a holiday. But even then, temper the amount you eat. A little bit of pleasure food gives the most pleasure because you will feel good afterwards.

Beware of rewarding yourself for small or regular accomplishments. Here's an analogy I bring up to my patients: if you train a dog to get a reward for doing a task, the dog will learn the task very fast.

Yet, dogs look and act healthy when they eat a small volume of dog food once per day. When you start showing love to your dog by feeding it from the dinner table and through the day, commonly and repetitively, you fatten up your dog, who will eventually find it difficult to move. The dog becomes sluggish and super happy only when getting the reward.

And, of course, we train ourselves, too.

Bad food as a reward conditions the mind to want bad food.

Avoid repetitive splurges, even if they are far apart.

You may have tried to eat well Monday through Friday and then splurge on the weekend, the so-called "cheat days." This pattern may have worked for a while, but for most of us, such a repetition doesn't work over time.

Eating for pleasure repetitively and as a reward changes our physiology. Speaking of dogs, recall Pavlov's dogs. Many years ago scientist Ivan Pavlov rang a bell, then fed them. The food caused the dogs to salivate—and the salivation was measured. Pavlov then demonstrated that after repeated food-bell pairings, the bell alone would cause salivation. Salivation was a physiologic response to the stimulus of either the bell or food.

The problem with eating for pleasure at specified times or events is that the brain becomes conditioned for the pleasure. You do not want to condition the brain for pleasure. You want to experience it every step of the way as if you discovered it for the first time. If you were to plan to make love every Saturday night at 10 p.m. and followed that pattern week after week, the incredible experience of making love would become boring and unfulfilling.

Let moments of pleasure unfold as if each moment was a new experience. Do it when the timing is right.

Have you felt the Monday morning blues? Your physiology is barking at you. Have you ever made the connection between food and the blues? When you do, you'll find it easier to change.

If you eat "badly" repetitively, even just every weekend, you will go through physiological withdrawal on the days you don't eat badly. In other words, you will feel like crap for several days or a week. This creates a cycle that does not feel good. This is much like the behavior of an addict. To avoid the withdrawal, you eat badly more frequently.

When you realize that common or repetitive bad eating requires a period of withdrawal, you'll realize that it isn't worth it, commonly or repetitively. Try it and see.

> *Pay attention to the withdrawal symptoms after you stop eating bad food. Remember that's the experience awaiting you after eating bad food.*

Exercise portion control.

Portion control works, but for most of us, exercising this control is difficult. As a way to make it easier, try this:

- On one occasion, eat a small portion of the restaurant chocolate cake or steak or whatever, and on another, each the whole piece or more.
- Ask yourself one hour after eating each how you feel. Do you have energy to do something fun and rewarding? Or do

you feel stuffed and ready to hit the couch and fall asleep to mindless TV?

- Repeat this test with other foods many times—it's important to reinforce the feel-good/feel-bad feelings. That's awareness training. When you're in a restaurant and you love steak and you are served the best eight-ounce steak ever, will you eat the whole thing? Try the self-test once again; pay attention to how you feel one hour after eating when you stop at four ounces, and again when you eat the whole eight ounces.
- As I describe in more detail in "Chapter 9: Tools for Success," a portion about the size of the palm of your hand provides a good guideline for portion size. And it's handy.

Get comfortable wasting food.

The major difference between eating a small portion and overeating is how you feel one hour after eating. You've already paid for the food, so that doesn't change. You have already seen, smelled, chewed, and tasted the food, so that doesn't change. No one went hungry because you wasted the food. Nothing on the planet changes because you wasted the food. The only thing that changes is how you feel one hour after eating and by the next morning.

Portion control is key to eating for pleasure. Your body can tolerate that brief, limited quantity of food containing lots of saturated fat, salt, and sugar, provided you keep the portion small.

It's OK to eat for pleasure even if it's "bad" food. Your brain just needs to know the rules.

Pleasure eating should be neither common
nor repetitive. And it should be quality.

Eating for nutrients: Fueling and refreshing our bodies.

Our physical being needs nutrients to function properly. Therefore, when eating, ask yourself, "Does this French fry have any nutrients in it?"

The question *"Am I eating for nutrients?"* combines the concepts of digestion and the chemical balance in foods.

What are nutrients? Nutrients are chemicals in food that our body needs to function optimally. How do we know which chemicals allow our body to function most efficiently? We have the answer when we make the connection between food and how we feel. Again, follow your intuition as you try different foods and ways to eat. Do your own trial-and-error problem-solving.

Self-experiment.

What is digestion? We eat until we feel satisfied. Then our body breaks down the food's components into individual chemicals—the nutrients—that are absorbed through the intestine and carried by the bloodstream to various organs. This is a complex orchestra of events. No portion of this process operates individually.

Many things influence digestion, including our mood, how fast or slowly we eat, how much liquids we drink when we eat, and so on.

Every part of the above process is important to any healthful-eating game plan. It's important to smell food, chew and taste food, eat slowly, and consume solid food instead of liquid food. One chemical in some food can interfere with the absorption of another chemical. This is simply too complicated to plan out. So the best way to get adequate nutrients is to eat a variety of whole foods, preferably farm-to-table food.

In general, pick food containing nutrients
and eat a variety of nutritious food.

Every meal, ask yourself if you are eating for nutrients, pleasure, or an unmet need.

Be aware.

To learn more about nutrient food, see Chapter 11: Becoming Your Own Nutrition Expert. Eat nutrient-smart, because nothing will make you feel better faster.

Tools for Success—Changing Your Eating Habits, Changing Your Life

CHAPTER 9

T
he only proven way to achieve long-term weight loss is to change eating habits.

I've seen such changes work in my many years of conversations with my patients, hearing their struggles and seeing how they've overcome those struggles by establishing new habits. Think of the following recommendations as eating "actions" that must be repeated to become habits. The beauty of these recommendations, however, is that they are simple, straightforward, and *doable*.

And remember that these actions are suggestions, guidelines, and best practices. Every day, ask yourself how well you did in sticking to these habits. That's the core of setting yourself as the goal and finding the solution to weight loss within yourself.

So never beat yourself up when you don't do as well as you need to. If you slip a bit, ask yourself how you can do better tomorrow. Have these self-conversations daily for the rest of your life, and you'll gradually begin to feel like the real you once again. You will achieve the goals of the feel-good diet. You'll exercise one hour power.

Solid eating habits + nutritional awareness = the real you.

Learning the nutritional value of food is important, but first focus on changing your approach to eating. Becoming your own nutrition expert is a matter of educational awareness, but if you don't follow these basic eating habits, you will limit your success.

As I discuss the following success habits, I'll explain the reasoning behind each one, and I'll recommend tools to accomplish them. Changing habits is complex, and we need tools for every complex task. Use the tools—use them repeatedly, so that they become everyday. Repetition creates a new habit naturally.

Remember: When you resist taking the actions recommended here, ask yourself the *million-dollar* question: "If I were given a million dollars to do this success habit today, would I do it?" Perform this exercise every time you feel the resistance, and repetition will make it a habit.

Commit to these success habits. Then chip away at making them the path of least resistance. Practice these processes—and invent a few of your own. *Make weight-loss artfully yours.*

Success Habits That Will Allow You to Change Your Life and Rediscover the Real You!

The weight-loss success program involves these practical, doable, effective habits, which I will cover point by point:

- Learn what fullness feels like, so you can avoid becoming over-full.
- Get comfortable wasting food.

- Learn the rapid and frequent grocery-shopping technique.
- Avoid unplanned eating.
- Eat every three to four hours.
- Eat soon after awakening.
- Learn to eat slowly.
- Don't drink with your meals.
- Limit drinking non-water liquids in general.
- Drink sufficient water when not eating.
- Limit refined table salt.
- Keep your body moving.
- Create good sleep patterns.
- Avoid the bathroom scale.
- Remember that feeling like the real you is the goal.
- Commit. Do. Celebrate.

"Duh! Tell me something new," you say? Well, read on and see if you get a new perspective.

Learn what fullness feels like, so you can avoid becoming over-full.

What's your favorite *over-indulgence* food? Think of it for a moment. Visualize the food on your plate. Can you smell it? Can you taste it? Savor the pleasure? Now chew and swallow. And have another bite. And another. But when does it stop? When all the food on the plate is gone?

What would be different if we stopped eating before we were *over-full*? Would the rotation of the earth change? Would more children in Africa starve? Would it cost less?

Nothing changes except how you feel one hour after eating.

It's your choice, and how you choose will determine how you feel one hour after eating and ultimately whether you have the energy and mental clarity to share your unique gifts with the universe.

When food tastes good, we tend to keep eating until it's gone.

The one-more-bite mentality drives us to over-eat.

The problem is that we have been over-eating for such a long time that most of us have lost the sensation to know what proper fullness is. "Satiety" is when you have eaten and are no longer hungry. In other words, you are satisfied. .

That *one-more-bite* mentality keeps us eating beyond satisfying hunger.

> *Unlike what the dogma dictates, we don't burn calories.*
> *We eat and digest food.*

Digestion breaks the food into chemical nutrients, which our bodies use in various chemical reactions. The paths these chemical nutrients take determine whether our body goes into energy-saving reserve mode or energy-expending mode. I believe that learning proper satiety is the most important habit to develop.

When we starve our body, it goes into energy-saving mode. When we eat to proper fullness, our body goes into energy-expending mode— which, I believe, is the signal that determines which path within the body that the food nutrients take—energy-conserving or energy-expending. And even if this theory is wrong, eating to the proper fullness translates into feeling energetic instead of feeling stuffed and ready for the couch.

Protein and fat gives us the most satiety. Protein seems to give us a more immediate sensation, and fat seems to be longer-acting. Both fit well into the equation of proper fullness. *Start your meal with protein* and savor it. Eat a few bites slowly and stop. Pick protein that has some healthy fat built in, like fish, or eat some veggies with healthy oil like avocado, coconut, or olive oil on it.

The volume and weight of food is as important as picking the foods that give you the most satiety. Believe or not, how much your food weighs tells you more about how much you should eat than the number of calories in food, or some blood-sugar statistic like the "glycemic index."

The One Hour Power pathway to your personal weight-loss success:
One hour after eating, ask yourself how stuffed you feel in the pit of your stomach. You should feel nothing. If you feel stuffed at all, think back to the volume of food you just ate and visualize what portions that are 25% smaller would look like. Embed this mental picture in your memory banks and recall it the next time you eat.

The phone app associated with this book—"One Hour Power"—will helpyou become aware of the volume of food that makes you feel the best.

Your hand is a good estimate of serving size. Sorry for the pun, but "it's handy." Also, hand size is proportionate to body-frame size.

Consider the palm of your hand up to the first knuckle as one serving size, two palms = two servings, and three = three.

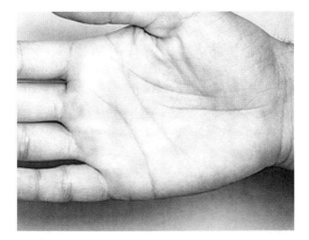

Ask if the food you just ate spread normally on a plate would equal one, two, or three palms. Then, one hour after eating, check in on your fullness.

Get comfortable wasting food.

Whether a habit engrained from our parents telling us to clean our plate or our genetics telling us to eat when we can, eating everything before us is a strong habit that's difficult to break. But you must break it—because there's no other practical way to achieve success.

Learning what fullness feels like and stopping—no matter how much food is on the plate—requires us to get comfortable wasting food.

Learn to throw away perfectly good food. For example, say you decide to keep all snack food out of the house. But somehow a bag of your favorite cookies made it home. Eat one serving and throw the rest away. That's one of the ways to give our brain what it wants when some unhealthy food makes it home or into our work environment, and still maintains a balanced weight. Our brain does not like when it subconsciously gets the message that it can't have something. The trick is to tell the brain that it can have the food, with some rules.

You must get comfortable wasting food
to achieve long-term weight management success.
This is one of the most important tools to learn. The best way to see if it's powerful is to try it several times. When you realize you can throw away good food and feel good, life changes.

Let me give you an example. I rarely eat apple pie, but I love it. So I was at this amazing grocery store and this large apple pie was sitting there in front of me, calling my name. I knew it was high-quality, so I bought it, took it home, put a piece in the microwave, and slightly warmed it. Then I dove in. I had two pieces. Then I did something that may make you say, "I can't do that." Keep in mind that the pie cost 25 dollars. But I threw it away. You know why? Because I knew that if I did not throw it away I would eat piece after piece until the whole pie was eaten. And then I would feel physically and mentally pissed at myself. I would feel like crap. But I felt good because I am comfortable wasting food. My mind really, really wanted that pie. And I gave my mind and body what they wanted, with some boundaries. I said to myself, "I can have it, but after I indulge in a couple pieces, it goes in the trash." My subconscious tells my inner brain, "You can have it, but there is a price to pay." If the food is of high quality, eating it may be worth it, provided you don't do it often or repetitively.

The One Hour Power pathway to your personal weight-loss success:
Reassert your commitment to success. Then commit to following the rule of getting comfortable wasting food. Purposely buy your favorite snack food and bring it home. Eat one serving and throw the rest away. Do this at least three times—you'll see that it works, for cost reasons, if nothing else.

Purposely over-eat your favorite restaurant food and ask yourself one hour after eating how you feel. Then, several days later, do it again, but stop at one-third of the previous amount—waste two-thirds. Again, ask yourself how you feel one hour after eating.

Use the "One Hour Power" app to refine this analysis.

Learn the joy of rapid and frequent grocery shopping.

Adhering to success habits is difficult without good-quality, nutritious food available. The best food to eat is whole foods and grass-fed or free range lean meat. They taste good only when fresh. If you eat a banana that's a little old, you will not want to eat a banana again any time soon. If you eat an avocado that has over-softened and turned brown, your taste for avocados fades. If you eat a carrot that has wilted, you will forget about carrots as a staple food. Such bad experiences erode a good habit.

We think of grocery shopping as a big chore event. We go up and down the aisles and fill up our cart. Then, when we get home, we have to unpack it all—and that takes time. Even the thought of that big chore is a huge obstacle to success.

Try the least-effort way first. Instead of planning a special grocery shopping time, just run into a grocery store on your way someplace. Set your timer for 15 minutes. Now, your job is to be in and out in 15 minutes.

Go to the produce section of the store. Get 10-15 items. Try two avocados, two oranges, an apple, spinach, celery, grape tomatoes, two bananas, some goat cheese, and some thin-sliced turkey breast. Head to the express lane and out the store.

Now, carry that bag of food everywhere with you. If you are in the car, the bag should be in the car. If you are out of the car, the bag should be with you. Then, every three to four hours, reach into the bag and eat a few items. One hour later, ask yourself how you feel. Then, realize how little effort it took to feed yourself and how amazing fresh food tastes.

Fresh food needs very little preparation. It tastes good as it is. Keep a knife in the bag to cut the avocado and anything else, as well as a spoon or fork. If you go to the store every couple of days, the food you buy is fresh, and you'll need only a small quantity of it. Because you're buying only a small amount, the shopping is fast—often faster than waiting in a fast-food line. Try and see for yourself.

Try to sense the energy in the produce part of the store. Does it feel good? Compare the feeling to less feel-good energy in your day. If you realize that it feels good to be in the produce section, you might want to go more often, to get a jolt of good energy. This may seem a little weird. Just be open to feeling it, and try it.

Most of the produce can be easily put in a bag or purse without a special container or preparation. As you learn the habit, you will probably want to get a special bag to carry your food. As a result, eating every three hours becomes not only easy but also tasty. And best of all, you feel good.

The One Hour Power pathway to your personal weight-loss success:
Try rapid and frequent shopping three or four times in a month, and observe how efficient and easy eating becomes. Once you realize this is easy, you'll be well on your way to success—because your brain likes easy. Life will get in the way of this new way to eat. As long as you realize that it works and you feel better eating this way, you will keep coming back to it. Time and repetition will form a new habit.

Avoid unplanned eating.

Snacking is unplanned eating. That doesn't mean that you have to stop all eating between meals, because I don't consider a small mid-day *something to eat* a snack—as long as it is planned.

Plan your meals and follow your plan. I have been a certified scuba diver since 1972. One of the key concepts of safe and successful diving is to *plan your dive and dive your plan.* This approach also applies to long-term healthy, feel-good weight success. In scuba diving, following the plan saves lives. Following this eating plan may save your life as well.

We live in busy times, and when and what we eat is often a last-minute thought. Haphazard eating promotes poor eating choices, which zap our energy.

This *stop-unplanned-eating mindset* eliminates the sneaky habit of snacking or grazing on food. These small amounts of nibble food add up over time and translate into extra pounds that our bodies find difficult to carry. This habit must be eliminated for success.

No snack food = no snacking.

Empty your house, car, and workspace of all but whole foods and lean meats. This is by far one of the best tools to avoid snacking.

The One Hour Power pathway to your personal weight-loss success:
Don't let food touch your fingers unless it is a planned mealtime. Each time food touches your fingers, ask if it was planned, and second, why you are eating—nutrients, pleasure, or an unmet need like love, or lack of fulfillment.

If snack food makes it into your house, eat one helping, enjoy it without blame, and throw the rest away. That desire to bring home the cookies, ice cream, or whatever disappears quickly if you can commit to this rule. If you want an apple pie bad enough to eat one slice and throw away the rest, go for it, because you won't keep doing it.

If you crave some snack food enough to get in your car, drive to get it, and then eat only one serving, the craving will disappear over time—I promise. The expense and the bother will help drive the craving away.

Eat every three to four hours.

You might think that there's only a thin line between grazing on food throughout the day and eating five to six times a day, yet the line is huge and significant.

"Eating every three to four hours" fits well with the guidance of learning what proper fullness feels like and planning your meals. Our digestion has a rhythm. We don't scientifically understand much of what's involved in the rhythm, but we know how it feels. And eating to proper fullness about every three to four hours seems to be the proper time span to avoid hunger pangs. Three hours is probably better than four, but four is a more manageable effort for most.

Get to know *your* schedule. Most people need something to eat mid-morning, mid-afternoon and possibly mid-evening. Plan these intervals, and between-meal eating becomes OK. Better yet, set your alarm to go off every three to four hours during the day.

Plan your regular meals and stick to that part of your eating plan as well. No skipping meals. Believe it or not, skipping meals blocks weight-loss success just as much as snacking. I've observed this in my patients over many years, and I can't fully explain it. But on a basic level, eating regular meals prevents us from getting too hungry, eating too fast, and over-eating.

If you begin to listen to your body, you will most probably find that when you eat a palm-size of food, you feel your best. When you eat that amount of food, you must eat every three to four hours, or you will get too hungry, make bad choices, and eat too fast.

Does our metabolism function better eating this frequently? I don't know, and no one else does either, because it is too hard to conduct a proper science experiment to prove one way or the other.

The concept of "we must eat to lose weight" seems counterintuitive. It seems far more intuitive that if eating causes us to gain weight, then not eating should help us lose weight. Yet, the information about eating that has been proven over and over again is that *starvation diets do not work.*

The One Hour Power pathway to your personal weight-loss success:
Set your mobile phone alarm to alert you every three to four hours during the day. When it goes off, eat something, *hungry or not.* This something can be as simple as an apple, a piece of string cheese, a handful of almonds, or a protein bar. Keep such edibles like this close by. Don't keep non-nutritious snack food close. (Nutrient food contains natural chemicals, not man-made chemicals.) It's important to eat, even

if you're not hungry. Establishing a regular eating schedule reinforces this healthy habit.

If you miss a meal, get super-hungry, and over-eat, laugh at yourself and ask how you can do better tomorrow.

Eat soon after awakening.

During a full night's sleep, our bodies have been in energy-conservation mode for hours. When awakening, our bodies need a signal that the nutrients that expend energy are again available. It doesn't take much food to deliver that signal.

The problem is that we think that breakfast—which recharges us— is a full meal deal at the local pancake house. The words we use affect us. So forget about the *breakfast* word. Just eat something soon after awakening. For instance, a handful of blueberries and a boiled egg will work, or maybe even just a handful of blueberries and later a protein bar, about mid-morning.

The One Hour Power pathway to your personal weight-loss success:
Before you go to bed, consider what you might eat when you wake up.

When you grocery shop, buy whole foods that you can eat quickly and easily first thing in the morning. (And by the way, most packaged breakfast cereals are junk food.)

Also, consider drinking eight ounces of water immediately upon awakening. I believe this signals to the body that all is well and gives the body permission to expend energy. The other advantage is that when we awaken, we are a little dehydrated.

Learn to eat slowly.

An important key to long-term weight-loss success is properly digesting food so that nutrients are available with the proper signals to keep our body in balance.

Weight gain = body out of balance.

We must eat slowly in order to allow our body to properly digest our food. Digestion begins much earlier than you think—when we see and smell food. Immediately, chemical messages are sent to the digestive tract and brain. Similarly, the body sends messages to the digestive system when we taste the food, and when we begin chewing and swallowing, in order to crank up the mechanisms that digest the food. Digestion takes time before your body sends you the sensation of fullness.

You see, the stomach is like a balloon. It doesn't have a fixed volume that it can hold. It's not like a metal container. Also, it doesn't stretch easily. What happens is it becomes insensitive to stretching from the "one more bite" mentality. The stomach has stretch receptors in it. For example, when we do weight-loss surgery on a morbidly obese person and remove part of his or her stomach, the common conception would be that that person has a really big stomach, because he or she can eat so much. But that stomach size is the same as the stomach size in a non-morbidly obese person.

The One Hour Power check-in will help teach your stomach to become more sensitive to fullness, so that you will feel full and satisfied on a small volume of food. It takes time and repetition to develop this sensitivity.

Sometimes we're busy and have minimal time to eat. And sometimes we're super hungry, and eating fast is the quickest way to satisfy the hunger. But mostly we eat fast out of habit.

People-watching is fun, so watch people eat and observe how often they chew food and have the next bite loaded on their fork, ready to enter the mouth as soon as they swallow. It's as if it's a gun that's locked and loaded to fire its first round as fast as possible.

Take time to enjoy your food. Your body will appreciate it.

We eat fast as if food were a gun locked and loaded for rapid fire.

The One Hour Power pathway to your personal weight-loss success:
Put down your eating utensil after each bite. Whether your fork, your spoon, or your hand, let go. Oddly, you will feel a sense of relaxation. It will feel like school recess. We digest better when relaxed.

If the *letting-go technique* doesn't slow you down, switch your eating hand to your non-dominant hand. Right-handers, wield the fork with your left hand, and vice versa. Your lack of practice with the other hand will slow you. This has the added advantage of helping you become ambidextrous. So, if for some reason you must learn to use your non-dominant hand better, begin eating with it.

Don't drink with your meals.
We don't need extra fluid to eat and digest food. We produce about two gallons of saliva each day, and our stomach produces about half a gallon of fluid each day.

Drinking with a meal is a habit and a tradition, not a necessity. It becomes a problem if we drink glass after glass with each meal. The excess fluid disturbs normal digestion, because it washes the food out of the stomach too quickly. Normal digestion requires the food to be in the stomach for 20 minutes.

Have you ever seen an eating contest? The winners drink lots of water as they eat. This washes the food into the small intestine, which can hold a large volume, because it is 22 feet long. However, that food is not properly digested and makes the winner feel, well, like crap.

Drinking a few sips with a meal is not a problem. But if you drink more than a few sips, it's time to change. Restaurants make changing this habit difficult because keeping the customer's water glass full is considered good service—and, of course, they encourage the sale of other drinks both soft and hard, because that's where their biggest profit margin lies. Servers will bug you to death if you have no glass next to your plate. And refusing the "good service" gets a little old every time you eat out.

So beware, and use your motivation to avoid drinking. Psychological experiments tell us that motivation is a short-term solution. This is a short-term event, so motivate yourself to drink only sips.

Because water enters and empties from the stomach very rapidly, you can drink liquids before you begin eating, and again about 15 minutes after you finish your meal.

The One Hour Power pathway to your personal weight-loss success:
When eating, bring no liquids to the table—water, soda, alcohol, whatever. If you need a drink so bad that you're willing to walk from your plate to the kitchen, then stand there and get one drink each time you feel the need, then do it. Commit to this trick and the habit will fade.

Limit eating out at restaurants to special occasions, and don't worry about it. If you must eat at restaurants frequently because of work or family obligations, ask the million-dollar question each time you drink. "Could I go through this meal without drinking more than sips if I were given a million dollars to do it?"

Limit drinking non-water liquids in general.
We live in the smoothie generation. Yes, we can pick some nutrient-dense food and throw it in a blender and rapidly drink it. And that concoction will give us the immediate feeling of fullness.

But smoothie-lovers don't realize that consuming "nutrient drinks" doesn't complement the built-in digestive process. Liquids are meant to hydrate our bodies. The liquids we drink enter the gastrointestinal tract and rapidly make their way to the small intestine, where they're quickly absorbed. In making a smoothie, we ask the blender to do the first phase of the work that our body normally performs, but the blending is only part of the stomach's 20-minute digestive process. Blending may bypass millions of bodily actions.

When we try to bypass nature's natural flow, we tend to screw it up in some way. For example, I have tested numerous athletes who subscribe to the thought that they must drink at least 100 grams of protein liquids a day. Yet, when their urine is tested for amino acids, deficiencies are usually revealed. One factor that explains this is that the protein doesn't have the adequate exposure to stomach acid needed to be properly integrated into the system. And there are probably many more reasons yet unknown. You see, when you chew and taste protein, your senses send signals downstream for the digestive process.

We think of liquid calories as soda, alcohol, and the like. We think of orange juice and milk as healthy drinks. Yet, they too are liquid food. Infants do well with liquid food because their digestive tracts are much different than those of the rest of us. Infant stomachs do not produce or contain acid. That's a good thing because the way they handle being over-fed is by regurgitating or spitting up. If the stomach had acid, it would burn the esophagus. Infants need liquid food, the rest of us need to see, smell, chew, and taste food.

If you can put something in your hand and it pours through your fingers, it is a liquid, and it will pour through your body almost as quickly. Drink food only on limited occasions.

We should eat an orange, not juice it.

Drinking smoothies may work well for you. If it gives energy and mental clarity, then it's good. *You should do what works for you.* Just don't be fooled into thinking it's the healthiest digestive way to get nutrients.

The One Hour Power pathway to your personal weight-loss success: If the liquid food you're about to consume is anything other than water, ask yourself, *Are you doing it for pleasure, and if so, do you do it commonly or repetitively?* If the answer is *yes*, resist drinking it.

Drink sufficient water when not eating.

Sometimes when we think we're hungry, we are, in fact, thirsty. Water may be the simple answer.

How much water do we need? Have you heard that you need to drink eight eight-ounce glasses of water each day (64 ounces, or a half-gallon)? None of these dictates are necessarily true. There's no good scientific study to support those recommendations. *Surprise! More dogma from poor science.* But there is a good method of observation and better testing.

We get water from the air we breathe, the food we eat, and the fluids we drink. The amount of water in the air varies and is measured by humidity. If you live in a high-humidity climate, you can drink less water. If you live in a dry, hot climate, you must consume lots of water.

But how do you know how much is enough? In general, if you urinate every three hours, and your urine is relatively clear, you're getting enough water. Of course, this guideline assumes that you are healthy and that your water-balance mechanisms are functioning normally.

A scientific way to know how much water is enough is to check your urine's "specific gravity" with a specific gravity refractometer (which you can buy online). The higher the specific number, the more the body needs water. A specific gravity of 1.010 suggests a normal water balance. A specific gravity of 1.035 suggests significant dehydration. You can measure urine output with a catheter in the bladder like you may have seen in a hospital. The normal adult urine output is 0.5cc/kg/hour. So, for a 180-pound adult, that would be about 40cc per hour—just a little more than a shot glass. So, every three to four hours would be in the range of a six-to-eight-ounce glass of water. If you need to urinate every two hours, you may be over-drinking.

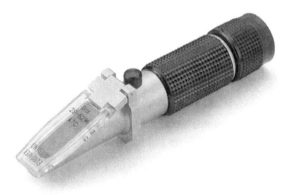

I don't expect you to go out and buy a refractometer, but using one may be a fun learning experience. Just know there is some science in observing whether you're urinating every three to four hours and whether it is relatively clear.

The One Hour Power pathway to your personal weight-loss success:
When you feel hungry between your planned times to eat, ask yourself how long it's been since you urinated. If it's been more than three hours, drink a glass of water.

Limit refined table salt.

Finding out if you're sensitive to refined salt and whether salt is affecting how you feel is simple. Use the trial-and-error method and find success in feeling better, quickly.

Eat salt-free through the week, Monday through Friday. Weigh yourself Friday morning as you awaken. Rate how you feel. Then eat your favorite salty meals Friday and Saturday. On Sunday morning, weigh yourself and rate how you feel. Have you gained a few pounds? Do you feel puffy and foggy-headed? Are your ankles a little swollen?

Refined salt is almost all sodium chloride—about 98%. Other food additives contain other types of sodium (look these up on ingredient labels), such as sodium benzoate, sodium nitrate, and monosodium glutamate (commonly known as MSG, which is often in processed foods). Many people don't respond well to refined salt or the sodium additives. Try and see for yourself.

Yet, our bodies need sodium for proper nutrient absorption and for proper nerve and muscle function. It's very important in how the kidneys maintain water balance.

Balance is the key word. Refined salt is not balanced; it is chemically altered. And as with most times when we manipulate nature, it does not work.

Whole foods have a natural balance of sodium. Himalayan and Celtic salt have a natural balance of minerals—usually around 80 different minerals, and sodium makes up about 50% of the mix. The salts that have a color to them most likely have not been bleached or refined.

Speaking personally, I am salt-sensitive and I avoid refined salt. I use Himalayan salt (again, check online for it), because it seems to work well for me. I use it as a condiment. I notice no swelling with it. I found this success through the trial-and-error approach. Again, try it and see for yourself.

Refined salt has small amounts of added iodine, which I believe is a very important and underused nutrient. To replace it, I take one tablet of iodine supplement every day. In my opinion, almost everyone should supplement iodine, even if eating table salt. Iodoral 12mg daily is a good source of iodine/iodide. Lugol's solution is another choice.

The One Hour Power pathway to your personal weight-loss success
Use the trial-and-error method to see how refined salt affects you. Each time you eat a salty food, ask if the taste was worth the morning-after feeling. Also, try Himalayan salt.

Keep your body moving.

Most people, especially personal trainers, equate exercise with weight loss. But exercise is poor at helping us lose weight. I suspect that you know this is true, because we've all tried the exercise approach. We can easily visualize that the amount of sweat should equal the amount of pounds falling off. But day after day of stepping on the bathroom scale leads to disappointment and bewilderment. We look at the scale and ask why?

Sometimes the number of pounds increases, and some trainers tell their clients that they are gaining muscle. That's wrong. Very few can actually grow new muscle after the age of forty (and probably even younger). The muscle retains water as it gets pumped, which is OK. But the muscle doesn't grow new muscle cells.

Don't get me wrong. Exercise is excellent at improving our quality of life. It's easily within the top four or five things that can significantly improve your quality of life. It helps us become fit, relieves stress, and improves our core for better posture.

*Exercise is just as important as good eating habits to improve
your quality of life, but it is poor as a method to lose weight.*

Expectations are important. The problem with the dogma of
exercising for weight loss is we feel defeated when we don't see the results
from our efforts, and then we find it hard to continue.

Exercising is all about habit. Proper expectations help build habit.
Can you visualize yourself being able to run and play a sport with your
kids? It takes a long time of repetition before exercise becomes habit.
And it's worth it! It makes you fit to enjoy life more fully.

Weight gain is a symptom of a body out of balance. Our body
functions better if we keep it moving. The only exception is sleep. Our
body needs sleep—real sleep, and not drug-induced sleep. Exercise helps
us sleep.

*Our bodies must keep moving to
function normally and be in balance.*

The One Hour Power pathway to your personal weight-loss success
Understand that regular exercise is a part of rediscovering the real you,
but that it is *not* a weight-loss strategy in itself. Exercise to strengthen
your core, better your posture, relieve stress, and make you fit. Do this
and your body will respond.

With that in mind, the two most important tools for success through
exercise are these:

- Find the time of day that is least likely to be interrupted, when
  you can give exercise the priority it deserves. Ask the million-
  dollar question each time you feel the resistance to blocking
  the time.

- Build in some method of accountability. Find an exercise partner and agree to make each other accountable. If your partner doesn't show up, give him or her a hard time, every time.

Create good sleep patterns.

Your body requires good sleep patterns to be in balance. A body in balance handles pollution, stress, and sickness much better. It's one of the big four: breathe, drink water, eat well, and sleep. Without these four we die. Sustained excess weight loss requires good sleep patterns.

A few tips:

- Spend some money and make a bed that's comfortable. Good mattress, high-quality sheets, and pillow.
- Make your bedroom as dark as possible.
- Keep the bedroom very cool—around 68 degrees while sleeping.
- Stop all TV-watching, computer work, and smartphone activity for at least an hour before bed.
- Try to establish a pattern of when you go to bed to sleep and when to wake up.
- Try to get seven to eight hours of quality sleep.
- Avoid coffee and stimulants from early afternoon.
- Get some exercise, but do not exercise for a few hours before bedtime.
- Do not eat for at least a few hours before bedtime.

Avoid the bathroom scale.

The bathroom scale gives us more bad information than good. The best judge of how your body is changing is closely observing how things fit, like your jeans, or your bathtub, or your car seat belt. Those indicate true progress.

The bathroom scale can be misleading. Weighing daily is a useful tool for monitoring water balance. If the pounds rise overnight, you're retaining water, probably from salt or maybe from hormonal reasons, such as menstruation.

Certain medications, such as those that are known as "corticosteroids," cause us to retain water. In a hospital setting, we weigh patients daily to help us understand the water balance, not whether we think they have lost fat, muscle, or bone. Losing fat, muscle, and bone is a slow process that's physiologically impossible to occur over several days. People weigh less early in the morning because we are a little dehydrated.

*The scale often disappoints us. It just sits there pointing at
a number that does not correlate with our effort to lose weight.*

Again, having the proper expectations is important. If you're working hard at changing your eating habits, stepping on the scale and seeing that you've lost very little weight is disappointing and might make you want to quit. Even worse is seeing that you've *gained* weight.

Those inner voices of doubt start the minute you step on the scale.

On the other hand, trying on your skinny jeans and seeing that they fit will be an emotional moment that might bring tears of joy.

The One Hour Power pathway to your personal weight-loss success.
Throw away the bathroom scale.

Remember *You.*

When your motivation begins to slip, re-visualize your goal. Remember what it feels like to look good in a suit, or in a pair of slinky pajamas, or in an athletic or military uniform, or in skinny jeans, or—yes—even naked.

The One Hour Power pathway to your personal weight-loss success.
Respect yourself. You deserve it. And after all this hard work, you deserve it all the more.

Commit. Do. Celebrate.

Celebrate each moment of success. There are no mistakes if you learn from them. Learn from those moments where you did not do so well and turn your experience into success. Find what works for you and fit into those skinny jeans at last.

You can be you. It's worth more than a million dollars. It's your life.

Changing habits is complex, and we need tools for every complex task. Use these suggestions as tools to help you change your habits.

Change your habits, and your life will change.

Pitfalls to Success and How to Leap Over Them

CHAPTER 10

Awareness is the key to all change, and especially crucial is awareness of the pitfalls that can trap you as you work toward better health and weight loss.

Such pitfalls regularly come up in the thousands of conversations that I have with my patients, and many other traps are waiting to be discovered in your personal self-experimentation. So recognize the pitfalls I list below and deal with them if they fit your situation, while being aware of your unique obstacles.

Remind yourself of such traps often, and laugh at yourself when they reappear—and they *will* reappear—then ask yourself how you will do better tomorrow. If a behavior repeats, it will keep repeating until you learn that it doesn't work and wish to change it. On the other hand, positive repetition succeeds—you just need to keep the *One Hour Power* conversation with yourself active.

Here are the common obstacles that you can avoid with awareness, understanding, and dedication to your healthy self:

1. False indicators of success
2. Escape mechanisms and resistance to change
3. Being resigned to defeat
4. Not understanding your deep-down level of commitment
5. Rituals, routines, and traditions that work against you
6. Instant gratification
7. Frugality
8. Poor sleep habits
9. Fad diets

Let's examine each in more detail.

False expectations

Pay attention to the power of the cliché *Quitters never win*. And then pay attention to this truism: *False expectations promote quitting*.

If we put effort into something and expect certain results and the result doesn't materialize, we want to quit. Here are two frustration traps that often trip up people working toward health and weight loss:

- **Expecting quick results.** And here I'm not even talking about "instant results." Change takes time. And results take even longer. If you're changing your eating habits appropriately, you'll see and feel *incremental* success. As I've noted before, some say it takes 21 days to change a habit, but I like to think in terms of chipping away and getting better and better.
- **Believing in misleading measurements.** As we have seen, that's the problem with using calories to help us determine

what you should eat. And that's also the problem with weighing yourself and using pounds lost as an indicator of success. Both are scientifically inaccurate indicators of success. The best judge of how your body is changing is closely observing how things fit, like your jeans, or your bathtub, or your car seat belt. The best way to know how much energy you get from food is not from counting calories. It comes from checking in one hour after eating and asking yourself, "How much energy do I have?" Those are the indicators of true progress.

In particular, the bathroom scale can be misleading. Weighing daily is useful primarily for monitoring water balance. If the pounds rise overnight, you're retaining water, probably from salt or maybe from hormonal reasons, such as menstruation. Certain medications, such as those that are known as "corticosteroids," cause us to retain water. And at the opposite end of the spectrum, people weigh less in the morning because they are a little dehydrated.

In a hospital setting, we weigh patients daily to help us understand the water balance, not whether we think they have lost fat, muscle, or bone. Losing those bodily components is a slow process that's physiologically impossible to occur over several days.

Weighing doesn't tell us how much fat has been lost. In fact, there are no reasonable methods to know how much fat we are losing in comparison to muscles, bones, and other tissues. Currently, more technical methods—such as those known in the medical community as the CT scan and the DEXA scan—are probably the best methods, but they have pitfalls and are too expensive to use.

The bathroom scale points at a number that often creates a false sense that what you are doing isn't working.

Again, having the proper expectations is important. If we're working hard at changing our eating habits, stepping on the scale and seeing that we've lost very little weight is disappointing and makes us want to quit. Even worse is seeing that we've gained weight.

Those inner voices of doubt start the minute you step on the scale.

On the other hand, if you try on your skinny jeans and they fit, well, it's an emotional moment that might bring tears of joy. So throw away the bathroom scale. The additional benefit? Your house will weigh less.

The One Hour Power pathway to your personal weight-loss success.
Take note of how your body is responding to your efforts, but don't "measure" your progress in the traditional sense. Set a reasonable and important short-term goal: how much energy you have one hour after eating and the next morning. Improve this result, and feeling good and losing excess weight will ultimately follow in time. Pay attention to your ultimate measurement and your ultimate goals. Once you start paying attention and noticing positive change, you'll be more inspired to continue the challenge of changing your eating habits with a proper set of expectations.

Escape mechanisms and resistance to change

Our brain is very good at concocting reasons to avoid tasks or regimens that are difficult or painful or stressful. There's always something else to do, some different task or chore or entertainment. The new task allows us to dodge the difficulty, pain, and stress.

Become aware of your escape mechanisms. Do you, for instance, want to go find some junk food and eat it when stressed?

It's natural to resist change. If you try to change an old habit, you will feel the resistance. As you feel it, recognize the discomfort and recognize the escape mechanisms that will appear in your thoughts.

Say you need to clean your garage because you are about to sell your house and it's Sunday and you're the only one who can get it done. Since selling your home for a good price requires the garage to be clean and selling your house is an important event, then despite the resistance to doing it, you most likely will go clean it.

The key to overcoming resistance to change is knowing that it's always present in change and that getting beyond the resistance is the only way to change.

Feel the resistance and laugh at it. Recognize the escape mechanisms and laugh at them.

Know what it feels like to accomplish your goal. For example, what would it feel like to fit into your favorite clothes or be able to run and play with your kids? Recall these thoughts when you feel resistance and recognize the escape mechanisms. Then you will feel that it is worth it and the resistance will fade.

Use the million-dollar question to rapidly bring the value of change into perspective. If you could have a million dollars to eat only a palm-size portion of food every three to four hours, would that be an easy way to make a million dollars? Eating healthy creates a body in balance, and a body in balance is worth more than a million dollars.

The One Hour Power pathway to your personal weight-loss success:
Feel the resistance to change that triggers escape mechanisms and laugh at it. Recognize the escape mechanisms themselves, and laugh at them, too. And think of your commitment to wellness and vitality as an escape from a life that does not feel like your life purpose.

Being resigned to defeat

You are likely not proud of the way you look and feel now, and of how you came to the point where you want to change.

The "defeats" that you've experienced before can lead to some of the psychological challenges that people encounter when attempting to get healthier and to lose weight.

- **"I'm not good enough."** Remind yourself of why you want to change your life for the positive—playing with your kids, being more active, being a better friend. You're doing it for yourself, but you're also doing it for those people who are important to you. The people that are important believe in you, and therefore, you are good enough.
- **"I have never been successful."** Consider that perception honestly. Tally your successes and discard the word *never* from that thought.
- **"I can't change."** Really? You're working to improve your health and well-being at this very moment by exploring how to go about it. That in itself is change—just keep doing it.
- **"I slipped up by eating too much, and that shows that I'm doomed to failure, because I'm certain to slip up again."** I don't believe that there's such a thing as a mistake—as long as the "mistake" teaches us something that benefits us. And slip-ups are to be expected. They are how we learn.

The One Hour Power pathway to your personal weight-loss success: How do you defeat defeatism? Celebrate your decision to improve your life and everything that you've done to accomplish that goal.

Not understanding your deep-down level of commitment

Be honest with yourself. Do you truly want to stop living the current story of your life? Are you ready to promise change?

A goal is an intention. You intend for it to happen. A promise is a full-blown commitment.

Imagine saying to your loved one before marriage that you have the goal of being monogamous. How well would that work?

If you're not ready to promise, you're not ready for change. Your reasons for feeling better and losing weight aren't important enough to commit to sustainable long-term change. As long as you like your day-to-day eating habits more than the results of changing those habits, you won't change, and all of this is a waste of time and energy.

The One Hour Power pathway to your personal weight-loss success:
Be honest with these questions: Is your current level of energy, mental clarity, and how your body feels holding you back from a life fulfilling your passions? Are you ready to leave the past? I believe that deep down, you're ready for change. You must believe it as well.

Rituals, routines and traditions that work against you

Your routines must change if you want to change your life. You must find new routines that work and stop the routines that don't work. Routines that don't work undermine your wellness goals can take various forms.

- **Daily eating habits and patterns.** Maybe you've always had a big breakfast, a snack between lunch and dinner, and some buttered popcorn while watching TV in the evening. As we've seen, habits are hard to break, even after we become aware of them. One such habit is mindless eating. Haphazard eating and eating without thinking about what you are eating only cause problems and don't work. Eating is such an integral part of our lives that we do it unconsciously, often just because the opportunity presents itself. The "See Food" diet. Think about what you eat. As long as you always have the self-to-self conversation about what you're eating and why you're eating, you will change.

- **Traditions.** *"My family always had mashed potatoes and gravy when serving beef."* What if you also ate too much mashed potatoes, or what if the family gravy is too rich and fatty? *"I always have coffee with breakfast."* What if the coffee makes you a bit jittery instead of waking you up, or what if you wash away the nutrient value of the breakfast with the liquids you drink? (That's why I advise against consuming liquids when eating.) *"We always serve grandma's cheesecake recipe when guests visit."* What if the cheesecake is too fatty, or you just plain don't like cheesecake? *"It's a holiday tradition."* Make eating foods that cheer you and energize you a new tradition—then you can truly celebrate.

- **Cultural and ethnic foods.** Honor your heritage, but be aware that some of the foods you "inherited" can cause you discomfort, weight gain, and maybe even bodily distress. Explore alternative ways of preparing the family dishes you have identified as problematic, and explore other dishes that characterize your heritage but that you haven't tried yet or have enjoyed little of.

- **Comfort foods.** As I discuss in Chapter 6: Committing to Changing Your Habits—Are You Ready , we often resort to eating food that makes us feel good *emotionally* instead of *physically.* Yes, we take solace in eating what Mom and Dad fed us on cold, rainy days, or after we didn't play so well in the soccer game. But take a different sort of comfort by eating food that energizes you and refreshes you after one of life's inevitable defeats or downturns.

- **Convenience foods.** Hectic schedules can lead to bad food choices—a quick burger from the drive-through if you're pressed for time, fatty frozen dinners if you're tired or running late and need to feed the family, and on and on and on. Keep healthy alternatives close by, including nonperishables that you can keep in your car or at work, and pre-cooked meals you can freeze and then reheat quickly. And as I've noted, a quick stop at the grocery store to buy fresh foods is often more efficient than waiting in line at the fast-food restaurant.

- **Pleasing those around you.** You know what makes you feel good, but your family hates certain of your favorites. What do you do? Prepare both—that's the most logical solution, but not always the most doable. Help those around you to understand your goals and gain their support for what you're serving. Share the *One Hour Power* method with your loved ones—perhaps they can benefit from it as well.

- **Social eating.** You go to a party and snack on the chips and the hors d'oeuvres, and you graciously accept a glass of wine you wouldn't otherwise have. Don't ignore what you've learned because you're "having fun" or feel obligated to indulge. And don't bypass your one-hour-after or next-morning analysis after social events.

- **Captive-audience meals.** In this category are business luncheons, conference or convention fare, community or organization banquets, charity dinners, and so on. You don't have much choice in what you're served, but you do have choices as to how much you eat, which specific parts of the meal you eat, and what you drink with the meal. Luckily, sponsors and caterers of such meals are increasingly aware of health and dietary concerns, which makes such eating easier.

The One Hour Power pathway to your personal weight-loss success:
You must find what works for you within any restrictions, obstacles, and challenges that you face, then make these techniques and practices a matter of habit. Repeating the habits that work over time and stopping

other habits that work against you will build a successful, sustainable ritual that works.

Instant gratification

We're human, and we take pleasure in instant gratification. This translates to snacking, choosing foods that taste good over those that promote wellness, and the "this is so good that I will have one more bite" mentality. That's pursuing instant gratification while ignoring the delayed gratification of feeling good, refreshed, and alert.

The One Hour Power pathway to your personal weight-loss success:
Become aware—daily—of how what you eat *now* affects how you feel *later.* Learn to live not only in the moment but also in the future just minutes away, because the moments when you feel your best are the moments to live in.

Frugality

You want to take care of your financial well-being too, correct? The "waste not want not" mentality is generally wise and helpful, but not necessarily when it comes to eating. The frugality trap takes a number of forms.

- **Cleaning your plate.** There's nothing frugal about cleaning your plate if your plate has too much food on it. Frugality suggests that it is economical or a waste. It is a waste to eat more than your body needs. What is not economical is buying too much food or putting too much food on your plate. Realize that you don't like wasting food. Because doing that feels bad to you, use it as a tool to help you change. That's why you must purposely waste food. Your subconscious will rapidly teach you that the way to be frugal is to not put so much food on your plate because your subconscious mind likes to feel good, not bad.

- **Buying too much food.** This often results from not understanding how much you really need to enjoy a meal. Also dangerous is being impressed with two-for-one deals in the grocery store, being sucked in by coupons or advertised specials for items you wouldn't otherwise buy, or "money-saving" combos in restaurants. At home, stock only what you need in the immediate future.

- **Choosing bargain foods that aren't right for you.** Don't settle for a less-expensive food that doesn't make you feel good. If you keep your portions small, then the extra expense for quality food is minimal.

The One Hour Power pathway to your personal weight-loss success: Simply, get comfortable wasting food, and don't bring too much food into your life in the first place. Our subconscious brain does not like wasting food, and to avoid what it does not like, it will disregard the urge for buying and bringing home bad food. Just make it a rule that if "bad" food makes it home, you will eat one serving and throw the rest in the trash. If you buy too much and it gets old before eating it, throw it away. Only for a few days from the day of purchase do fresh whole foods taste good. If you eat old "healthy food" you will lose your desire to eat it. If you eat fresh food, you will want more.

Poor sleep habits

A recent article in *The Journal of Clinical of Endocrinology and Metabolism* (which I'm sure you keep on your coffee table) found that just one night of poor sleep can throw your appetite into overdrive, setting you up to overeat.

In fact, lack of quality sleep will affect every aspect of your life—sleeping well is an important element of the body's balance you are working to achieve in order to feel good and healthy.

Here are some basics for getting a good night's sleep.

- **Before going to bed, spend a few minutes writing down your priorities for the next day**, but don't focus on solutions to problems. Tell your brain that you'll read your list in the morning and at that time you'll start working on solutions to getting it all done. You'll worry less and sleep better—and usually wake up with the solutions in mind.
- **Sleep in a dark, quiet, cool room.** Don't go to bed watching TV, and don't be around any bright light before going to bed.
- **Avoid caffeine after noon.** Coffee, energy drinks, and certain soft drinks are obvious sources of caffeine. But did you know that other sources include chocolate, pain relievers, and certain weight loss pills?
- **Avoid sleep "meds."** I'm not a fan of medicine sleep aids, though I have prescribed them many times. Using them is better than not sleeping at all. However, sleep meds will often prevent you from finding the balance and quality of life you desire.
- **Commit to regular sleep patterns despite circumstances.** For example, some work schedules make quality sleep difficult. Don't use such circumstances as an excuse to allow haphazard sleep patterns. Establish a consistent sleep routine.
- **Find ways to stop snoring.** If you snore, you probably have sleep apnea. If you have sleep apnea, you're not getting enough oxygen while sleeping, and you are not getting an adequate night's sleep. See a doctor and start using a breathing machine or other apparatus to sleep. Sleep apnea is a severe sign that

your body is out of balance, and the best way to resolve it long-term without sleep aids is to change your eating habits and lose some weight.

- **Watch the sun rise and the sun set.** Relax into the beauty of nature and the importance of the sleep cycle. Stay connected to nature and nature's rhythms.

The One Hour Power pathway to your personal weight-loss success:
As you log your reaction to foods using *The One Hour Power Diet* method, note those occasions when your sleep habits fell out of balance the night before. Research advice and best practices about sleep habits on the internet. Find what works for you.

Fad diets

Fad diet programs that involve severe changes present a danger to your results. An example is skipping meals—or, for that matter, any starvation method.

Skipping meals makes you too hungry, and by the time you eat, you will overcompensate. You will eat too much, and you will make poor food choices. When you eat a palm size or one serving of food, you will find you feel better after eating. If you eat that size of a serving, you must eat every three to four hours or you will get too hungry. There is no known science to prove how often you should eat, but experience and trial and error will teach you what works.

Starvation methods, such as very low-calorie diets, deplete the body of nutrients and throw the body more out of balance. They also cause more muscle loss than eating small meals every three to four hours. You need your muscles for posture, breathing, and many important functions. This concept doesn't need some big, expensive research to prove true. Look at anyone that follows the starvation method. Look at the shoulders, thighs, buttocks, and arm muscles. They look scrawny.

That person likely moves more slowly, and maybe more awkwardly. That person *looks* tired. This is a body out of balance. Just look and you will see.

Similarly, don't suddenly switch to eating only one type of food— the Twinkie diet mentioned earlier, as an extreme example. Again, you risk throwing your body out of balance and robbing it of nutrients. For example, when we go on a 1,000-calorie diet, which is usually nutritionally depleted, we lose weight—and then we regain all the weight back plus 10% on average. Because the diet is based on calories, we often avoid foods that have nutritional value but too many calories. As we become nutritionally depleted, our body becomes more out of balance. The more out of balance your body is, the more years it will take to get it back in balance.

The One Hour Power pathway to your personal weight-loss success:
Always remember the keyword that connects your food with your life: *balance.* You must balance timing, food types and portions, and lifestyle. When you do, you'll come a long way in "Becoming Your Own Nutrition Expert," our next and final chapter.

CHAPTER 11

Becoming Your Own
Nutrition Expert

There are so many ways to learn, including in a formal setting such as a classroom with a teacher. You can also learn by observing, experiencing, reading, researching, and just doing, among other ways. I suggest becoming your own food expert by becoming your own teacher and then becoming your own best student. Learn from yourself. Learn from your experience.

When you can connect the dots between what you eat and how it makes your feel, you become your own best teacher about the lessons you want to learn. You set the ground rules for your own teaching.

Food is essentially about nutrition, but not always. The definition of nutrition is simple: "food that provides ingredients and chemicals that cause our mind and body to function." These ingredients and chemicals are called nutrients. And learning the individual nutrients that contribute to your well-being helps you to identify other foods that can lower, maintain, or optimize our health.

The problem that you will run into when searching for information about nutrition and the resulting advice, however, is that we don't know very much. And nutrition is simply too complex and expensive to study. It's too difficult to control all the variables so that you can show if you do "X" then "Y" will happen.

Some experts keep us confused with conflicting information. Recently, *The Annals of Internal Medicine* analyzed 72 studies and concluded that "there's just no evidence to support the notion that saturated fat increases the risk of heart disease," according to *The New York Times*. For years, experts have been advising against eating butter out of fear of saturated fat. Which experts are right?

It would be great if you could consult with someone who could give you a list of what foods made you feel good an hour after eating, the next morning, and year after year—what to eat in order to perform optimally and have a normal weight. However, such people do not walk in your shoes, wear your rings, or try to fit into your skinny jeans. Instead, the answer is within you.

Still, I agree with the general expert consensus that a balanced diet of unprocessed foods, and mostly plants, is best, and I'm certain that most experts agree with me that over-eating and sporadic, undisciplined eating can hurt your body and reduce your energy.

Read or listen to nutrition advice, and try it to see how it works for you. Learning is a process. The process of finding the right food for you comes through learning what works for you. But for the reasons I just listed, ultimately you must learn by experience. The bottom line is that it's up to you to provide and eat the food that causes your mind and body to function the way you want it to function—which is the Real You.

Currently I suggest these sources of good information to listen to and to try.

1. **NuVal (http://www.nuval.com/)**

    This is a scorecard of the nutritional value of food—one that's useful at the grocery store. It was developed by Dr. David Katz and a team of knowledgeable nutritionists. Some grocery stores are sharing this information, and more will in the near future. The 30-plus-factor algorithm that determines the NuVal score overcomes many of the inadequacies.

2. **ANDI (https://www.drfuhrman.com/library/andi-food-scores.aspx)**

    The Aggregate Nutrient Density Index is also a scorecard, and it is useful for understanding the nutritional value of plant source foods. It was developed by Dr. Joel Fuhrman. Instead of scoring grocery store food label information, it evaluates individual ingredients in food. The ANDI score is based on the micronutrients/calories. The pitfall is that the scoring uses calories in its calculations. As you know, I consider counting calories a very inaccurate way to measure food energy.

While both methods have pitfalls, Dr. Katz and Dr. Fuhrman have many years of experience and have very good advice. I suggest trying the foods that rank high on their scorecards to see how they work for you.

Self-experimentation with highly recommended foods is one way you will become your own nutrition expert. Be open to trying new foods, but be skeptical, as well. Let the food prove that you feel good—or not—when you eat it.

Listen to the teacher, and then learn by experience.

How to become your own teacher

You become your own teacher as soon as you start listening to your body and begin recognizing how food makes it feel. The following ways will also help strengthen you as a teacher and will help you become your own nutrition (food) expert:

1. Become aware of the ingredients and chemicals in your food and how they make you feel.
2. Learn about the chemicals in the food you eat. Conduct an internet search for the chemical name on the food label or via phone app and read about it. Learn why the chemical is in the food. Is it a product of industry or nature? Is it food or an additive? What is the purpose of the chemical?
3. Use your energy to learn about the foods you eat and gradually add variety. This is a more efficient use of your time and energy, in contrast to shopping for some new magical supplement.

Here are some basics that will help you along.

1. Rice, soy, wheat, and corn are major ingredients in most packaged food. These foods have been genetically changed to tolerate pesticides and to enhance transport and storage. They can be bagged and shipped to impoverished nations to keep poor people from starving. They are cheap survival foods. *Cheap* translates into better profit margins on packaged food found in the grocery store. In my opinion, these foods don't promote optimal well-being. Self-experiment and see for yourself.
2. Beware of information on the front of packaged food. That's marketing.
3. Some chemicals in food promote better absorption of some nutrients and some block the utilization of some nutrients.

For example, vitamin C helps the absorption of iron. Tea blocks the absorption of iron. You can search for this sort of information, yet the subject is simply too complex, and it's expensive to study. So what's known is a very small piece of the overall eating-right puzzle. The best way to get optimal nutrition is to eat a variety of foods that your body responds well to.

4. The most common foods that people have trouble with:

- **Gluten from wheat, barley, and rye.** It may come from the flour used to make the food or it may be an additive. Foods containing gluten include most bread, pasta and crackers, and many packaged foods.

- **Eggs.** Some people are sensitive to eggs, and eating them can result in skin problems, asthma, and nasal congestion. However, if eggs don't make you feel bad, I think they are one of the highest-quality sustainable protein sources and should be a major component of your diet.

- **Dairy.** That is, milk and cheese from a cow. Goat's milk is often tolerated well, and I think that it is one of the healthiest products because of its balance of calcium, magnesium, and phosphorus. Goat cheese contains sodium, which the body needs (and in this form can be well tolerated).

- **Refined table salt**, which makes many people's fingers and ankles swell. Try Himalayan or Celtic salt. Iodine is added to refined salt, yet it's a poor source of iodine. I recommend supplementing iodine/iodide instead. Go to Amazon.com and order Iodoral and take 12mg daily. Consult with your personal physician before supplementing if you suspect you are allergic to iodine. Do your own provocative test and see if you tolerate Himalayan or Celtic salt without retaining water and getting puffy.

- **Soy.** Many packaged foods include soy as a filler or an additive. It's also in tofu, edamame⊠, soy nuts, and soy milk, and it's used as an ingredient in many foods labeled as vegetarian. It was touted as a health food yet has never been proven to be healthy. It's hard to prove, but I think it's a poor-quality protein source as well. It also has estrogen-like effects.

- **Nuts.** These are a staple in my daily diet, because I feel good when I eat them. They contain many different chemical nutrients that may serve your body well. If you don't feel good after eating them, don't eat them. Many people are allergic and some are sensitive to peanuts and tree nuts. Consult with your personal physician if you suspect an allergy.

- **Animal protein.** Animals kept in an environment in close proximity to other animals—such as a feedlot or a crowded chicken coop—get sick unless they're treated with lots of medicines to keep them well. And supplements promote rapid growth of these animals, which translates into more profit. So some people that seem to be sensitive to some animal protein like beef may be reacting not to the meat but to the means used to treat the animals. I believe free-range grass-fed animal protein is good.

The Self-Discovery Process in Action

So how would the activities and the self-discovery I've described in *One Hour Power Diet* look in real life? Let's follow a hypothetical person through her day as her own nutrition expert.

Alice wakes up and drinks a large glass of water. After a morning bowel movement, she brews her morning cup of coffee or tea. She eats a small amount of food.

Later, she eats something out of her rapid-grocery-shopping bag—about every three hours. She drinks water often.

At each meal during the day, she asks herself why she is eating: for nutrients, for pleasure, or for an unmet need. She visualizes the volume of food she is eating and relates it to her palm size: one palm, two palms, or three palms. She photographs the food with *One Hour Power Diet* phone app or writes down details of the meal in a journal. She reads the food labels for chemical information about the food she is eating.

One hour after eating, Alice checks in and asks herself how much energy and mental clarity she has, and how well her body feels. She pays particular attention to the foods that cause common sensitivities.

That night, she conducts internet searches on the various chemicals that the labels have identified and learns about them. For example, she may have recognized previously that gluten made her feel bad, so she is trying to avoid gluten. She reads "tapioca" on the ingredient label of the gluten-free food she had at her meal. On the internet, she discovers that tapioca comes from the cassava root, primarily from Brazil. It's a product of nature, not an industrialized food. It's a pure starch with very little in the line of additional nutrients. She searches for starch and reads that it is a carbohydrate used for thickening and stiffening food and gluing it together.

Before bed, she writes down what she wants to accomplish the next day. She sleeps in a cool dark room without the TV on. She meditates three minutes before starting her day, and again in the evening before bedtime.

After a week or more, Alice reviews her information and becomes more aware of which foods and food combinations made her feel good and which ones made her feel bad. She pays particular attention to how the food volume affected how she felt one hour after eating. She also pays attention to how often she went more than four hours before eating and how that affected the choices she made and how she felt one hour after eating.

Alice has learned that she feels better when she eats food from nature, a palm-size of food, a portion every three to four hours, mostly plant food, and some animal protein that's grass-fed or from the wild.

Alice recognizes that she feels better when she drinks water through the day, requiring her to urinate roughly every three hours.

And over time, she recognizes that she's finally fitting into smaller clothes from the back of the closet. She finds herself doing the things she really loves because she feels good.

Alice finds that with good sleep, adequate hydration, and good eating habits, she finally feels like the Alice that was meant to share the amazing, unique gift of her soul and passion with the universe.

The Author

Dr. Cliff Thomas has been a doctor for three decades, starting as a general surgeon, then turning to his major interest and specialty—the control and treatment of obesity problems—known in technical terms as bariatric medicine. That practice is active and successful.

His previous e-book on weight-loss surgery success, *Skinny Jeans at Last: Secrets to Long-Term Weight-Loss Surgery Success*, has remained in the top 6 sellers among Kindle books on weight-loss surgery in the previous two years.

Dr. Thomas has been featured in a TLC documentary—"The Half Ton Mom"—in which another surgeon and he performed the largest gastric bypass in the world.

The One Hour Power Diet results from helping patients through the struggles of changing their eating habits. In seeing thousands of patients one on one, Dr. Thomas found that he couldn't give patients a list of eating rules and a list of healthy food that would apply specifically to them and allow them to begin eating well. Each patient had different circumstances, tastes, cultural eating habits, and struggles. He probed into their struggles and discovered why they resisted change. Then he learned how to help them give up the resistance and change their habits in ways that fit them. He also learned the true reason they wanted to lose weight: to feel like the person they knew was inside that overweight body. Often they would tear up as they spoke of *fitting into those skinny jeans.*

Previous Publications

- *Skinny Jeans at Last: Secrets to Long-Term Weight-Loss Success.* CreateSpace, 2011.
- *10 Reasons to Not Ignore Reflux or Heartburn.* CreateSpace, April 2013.
- Contributions to two books:
  - *No Mistakes! How You Can Change Adversity Into Abundance,* Madisyn Taylor, Sunny Dawn Johnson, and HeatherAsh Amara. Hierophant Publishing, June 2013. My chapter: "The Art of Taking the High Road."
  - *Breakthrough! Inspirational Strategies for an Audaciously Authentic Life,* Janet Bray Attwood, Marci Shimoff, Chris Attwood and Geoff Affleck. Turning Stone Press, Sept. 2013. My chapter: "The Art of Being Present in Difficult Situations."